FRCOphth Part 1

400 SBAs and CRQs

SECOND EDITION

FRCOphth Part 1

400 SBAs and CRQs

SECOND EDITION

Robert G Peden MBBS(Lond) MA(Oxon) FRCOphth
Consultant Ophthalmologist, Princess Alexandra Eye Pavilion
Honorary Clinical Senior Lecturer, University of Edinburgh
Edinburgh, Scotland, UK

H Nikki Hall MBChB BSc(Hons) FRCOphth
Consultant Ophthalmologist
Queen Margaret Hospital, Dunfermline
Fife, Scotland, UK
Honorary Clinical Tutor, University of Edinburgh
Edinburgh, Scotland, UK

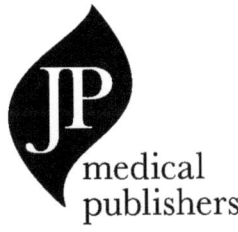

London • New Delhi

© 2024 JP Medical Ltd.
Published by JP Medical Ltd
83 Victoria Street, London SW1H 0HW, UK
Tel: +44 (0)20 3170 8910   Fax: +44 (0)20 3008 6180
Email: info@jpmedpub.com   Web: www.jpmedpub.com

The rights of Robert Peden and H Nikki Hall to be identified as the authors of this work have been asserted by them in accordance with the Copyright, Designs and Patents Act 1988.

All rights reserved. No part of this publication may be reproduced, stored or transmitted in any form or by any means, electronic, mechanical, photocopying, recording or otherwise, except as permitted by the UK Copyright, Designs and Patents Act 1988, without the prior permission in writing of the publishers. Permissions may be sought directly from JP Medical Ltd at the address printed above.

All brand names and product names used in this book are trade names, service marks, trademarks or registered trademarks of their respective owners. The publisher is not associated with any product or vendor mentioned in this book.

Medical knowledge and practice change constantly. This book is designed to provide accurate, authoritative information about the subject matter in question. However, readers are advised to check the most current information available on procedures included and check information from the manufacturer of each product to be administered, to verify the recommended dose, formula, method and duration of administration, adverse effects and contraindications. It is the responsibility of the practitioner to take all appropriate safety precautions. Neither the publisher nor the authors assume any liability for any injury and/or damage to persons or property arising from or related to use of material in this book.

This book is sold on the understanding that the publisher is not engaged in providing professional medical services. If such advice or services are required, the services of a competent medical professional should be sought.

Every effort has been made where necessary to contact holders of copyright to obtain permission to reproduce copyright material. If any have been inadvertently overlooked, the publisher will be pleased to make the necessary arrangements at the first opportunity.

ISBN: 978-1-78779-171-8

British Library Cataloguing in Publication Data
A catalogue record for this book is available from the British Library

Library of Congress Cataloging in Publication Data
A catalog record for this book is available from the Library of Congress

Publishing Manager:	Nikita Chauhan
Editorial Assistant:	Keshav Kumar
Cover Design:	Seema Dogra

Foreword

Gone are the days of long essay questions necessitating focused revision on a small number of topics. The subject matter contained in the modern FRCOphth Part 1 examination covers almost the entire syllabus, making it vital to ensure that revision covers the full breadth of the subject. By using this book to prepare for their examination, candidates will equip themselves with the knowledge and techniques necessary to pass.

Even though a very broad factual knowledge is required, there are many facts and figures that tend to pop up repeatedly in the examination questions (such as angles, thicknesses, volumes and percentages). The more that candidates practise with mock papers, the more conversant they will be with these specifics and the better prepared they will be.

Writing multiple choice questions is not an easy task, as examiners have to ensure that correct answers are incontrovertibly true and not just possibilities. They must also ensure distractors (the incorrect answer options) are not so obviously wrong that the question becomes too easy, or not so nearly right that they could, in fact, be right. A good examination multiple choice question (MCQ) must therefore be written with careful thought, and only by working through an extensive collection of such questions can candidates gain familiarity with the format, and confidence in their ability to answer them correctly.

Constructed response questions test knowledge across a range of scenarios. Thankfully, candidates for the FRCOphth Part 1 will have had some clinical experience and will have developed a broad working knowledge. Only with practice, however, will candidates become familiar with the topics commonly tested using this format. Again, this familiarity will help candidates to tackle these questions successfully by teaching them the importance of paying attention to detail, of reading questions carefully and of managing their time effectively.

The extensive explanation sections in this book not only provide in-depth reasoning behind the correct answers, but also provide candidates with a wealth of information relevant to the FRCOphth Part 1 examination. To pass this examination you must have clinical experience and you must know your facts. But, equally you must know how to pass. This book will give you the confidence and knowledge to achieve that goal.

Robert I Murray
Consultant Ophthalmologist and Head of Service
Borders General Hospital, Melrose, UK
Past Lead Ophthalmology Examiner, Royal College of Surgeons of Edinburgh
Ophthalmology Module Leader, University of Edinburgh, UK
November, 2015

Preface to the second edition

Since the publication of the 1st edition of this book we have been delighted by the feedback from colleagues and readers who have found it a useful aid for preparing to pass their FRCOphth Part 1 examination.

The examinations of the Royal College of Ophthalmologists are in a state of flux at the time of writing, brought about by the unprecedented challenges of the global coronavirus pandemic. The impact of social distancing and travel restrictions have accelerated a shift to digital proctored examinations, and alongside this the FRCOphth Part 1 examination has been reformatted into two multiple choice question (MCQ) papers, each of 90 questions and each lasting 2 hours.

At present it is unclear whether the shift to two MCQ papers is a permanent change. Constructed response questions (CRQs) are certainly compatible with digital proctored examinations, and indeed this format potentially facilitates the inclusion of high-quality images and investigations. CRQs were included in the early digital proctored examinations for the FRCOphth Part 1 examination, including the digital drawing of ray diagrams.

We have elected not to change the format of the book at present, for several reasons:
- It is possible that the examination format will continue to evolve following the pandemic, and at present this book is the only published source of sample CRQs
- The CRQs in this book cover a range of topics across the curriculum which are likely to appear in the current examination
- Many of the CRQ topics are of direct clinical relevance
- Answering CRQs requires a different use of knowledge and recall, and helps to cement an understanding of the topics which is complementary to the understanding gained by doing single best answer questions (SBAs)

In preparing the second edition, we have edited the contents to improve the clarity and accuracy of the questions and explanations, and to incorporate developments in the field. The essence of the book, which has contributed to the examination success of so many of our colleagues, remains unchanged. We hope you find it similarly useful, and wish you well with your studies and examinations.

Robert Peden
Nikki Hall
April, 2023

Preface to the first edition

In our experience the most high yield way to prepare for the FRCOphth Part 1 exam is to practise using high quality revision questions. Although there have been several sources of multiple choice questions available, none of these have included constructed response questions (CRQs). No longer! *FRCOphth Part 1: 400 SBAs and CRQs* provides targeted and structured preparation material for the entire FRCOphth Part 1 exam and is the only revision book with practice CRQs.

The examination comprises 120 single best answer questions (SBAs), which are in best-of-four multiple choice format, followed by 12 CRQs. The latter are multi-part short answer questions, typically working around a ray diagram, photo or clinical investigation. CRQs constitute half of the examination marks, so practice is essential in order to achieve a pass mark. The good news is that they are often clinically relevant and make for comparatively enjoyable revision.

The question layout in each chapter mimics the structure of the exam, with SBAs followed by CRQs. The questions are grouped by subject in the first two chapters to facilitate focused study, whereas the final chapter is unstructured. You may wish to use this as a complete mock exam. The questions presented here are deliberately skewed to the more challenging end of the spectrum. By tackling conceptually difficult topics that could and do appear in the exam, we hope that the actual exam will feel a lot more achievable. Do not be discouraged if you don't get questions right the first time. The feedback section, with its clear explanations, key diagrams and tables, will ensure you learn something worthwhile and make efficient use of your study time. We also recommend background reading from the publications listed in the bibliography.

This book has broad coverage of the FRCOphth Part 1 exam syllabus in one portable volume. We hope it will maximise your chances of examination success.

Nikki Hall
Robert Peden
November, 2015

Contents

Foreword	v
Preface to the second edition	vii
Preface to the first edition	ix
Acknowledgements	xii
Bibliography	xiii

Chapter 1 Exam Paper 1: Structured Practice Paper

Questions: SBAs	1
Questions: CRQs	23
Answers: SBAs	33
Answers: CRQs	71

Chapter 2 Exam Paper 2: Structured Practice Paper

Questions: SBAs	89
Questions: CRQs	110
Answers: SBAs	121
Answers: CRQs	157

Chapter 3 Exam Paper 3: Unstructured Mock Exam

Questions: SBAs	177
Questions: CRQs	197
Answers: SBAs	206
Answers: CRQs	240

Acknowledgements

Many people have given us to help, inspiration, material and advice while writing this book. We would like to thank all of our colleagues, and in particular the following people:

Ali Al-Ani, Consultant Ophthalmologist
Ana Maria Armbrecht, Associate Specialist in Ophthalmology
Shyamanga Borooah, Assistant Clinical Professor of Ophthalmology
Marion Brannan, Senior Medical Photographer
Mei-Ling Cheng, Consultant Ophthalmologist
Martin Galea, Consultant Ophthalmologist
Alan Patrick Gibb, Consultant Medical Microbiologist
Colin Goudie, Consultant Ophthalmologist
Sarah Jane Griffin, General Practice Doctor
David Hall, Wing Commander and Consultant Intensive Care Physician and Anaesthetist
Ashraf Khan, Consultant Ophthalmologist
Stephen Madill, Consultant Neuro-Ophthalmologist
Roly Megaw, Clinical Lecturer and Consultant Ophthalmologist
Robert Murray, Consultant Ophthalmologist
Mohammad Zuhair Mustafa, Specialty Registrar in Ophthalmology
Mark Rodrigues, Consultant Head and Neck and Neuroradiologist
Conrad Schmoll, Consultant Ophthalmologist
Andrew Tatham, Consultant Ophthalmologist and NHS Scotland Research Clinician
Hannah Timlin, Consultant Ophthalmologist
Naing Latt Tint, Consultant Ophthalmologist
Jonathan Whittle, Associate Specialist in Ophthalmology
Cameron Lowe, Specialty Registrar in Medical Ophthalmology

We are grateful for use of the following images, which have been reproduced with permission:

Chapter 2: Figure in CRQ question 1 (page 110) from Dada T, Sharma R, Sobti A. Gonioscopy: A Text and Atlas. New Delhi: Jaypee Brothers Medical Publishers (P) Ltd., 2013.

Chapter 2: Figures A and B in CRQ question 8 (page 117) from Boyd S, Boyd B. New Trends in Ophthalmology – Medical and Surgical Management. New Delhi: Jaypee Brothers Medical Publishers (P) Ltd., 2013.

Chapter 3: Figures A and B in CRQ question 1 (page 197) from Clarke LE, Clarke JT, Helm KF. Color Atlas of Differential Diagnosis in Dermatopathology. New Delhi: Jaypee Brothers Medical Publishers (P) Ltd., 2014

Chapter 3: Figure A in CRQ question 10 (page 204) from Public Health Image Library – CDC/J. Pledger (ID 3766)

Chapter 3: Figure B in CRQ question 10 (page 204) from Public Health Image Library – CDC/J. Miller (ID 14494)

Bibliography

Elkington AR, Frank HJ, Greaney MJ. Clinical Optics, 3rd edition. Hoboken: Wiley-Blackwell, 1999.

Forrester JV, Dick AD, McMenamin PG, Roberts F, Pearlman E. The Eye: Basic Sciences in Practice, 5th edition. Philadelphia: Saunders, 2020.

Snell RS, Lemp MA. Clinical Anatomy of the Eye, 2nd edition. Hoboken: Wiley-Blackwell, 1997.

Salmon J. Kanski's Clinical Ophthalmology: A Systematic Approach, 9th edn. Netherlands: Elsevier, 2020.

Sundaram V, Barsam A, Barker L, Khaw P. Training in Ophthalmology (Oxford Specialty Training), 2nd edition. Oxford: Oxford University Press, 2016.

Denniston A, Murray P. Oxford Handbook of Ophthalmology, 4th edition. Oxford: Oxford University Press, 2018.

Ferris J, Easty DL. Basic Sciences in Ophthalmology: A Self Assessment Text, 2nd edition. Hoboken: Wiley-Blackwell, 1998.

Guthoff RF, Katowitz JA. Oculoplastics and Orbit (Essentials in Ophthalmology). New York: Springer, 2006.

Rang HP, Ritter JM, Flower RJ, Henderson G. Rang & Dale's Pharmacology, 9th edition. Netherland: Elsevier, 2019.

Koeppen BM, Stanton BA. Berne & Levy Physiology, 7th edition. Netherland Elsevier, 2017.

Barrett KE, Barman S, Brooks H, Yuan J. Ganong's Review of Medical Physiology, 26th edition. New York: McGraw-Hill Medical, 2019.

Yentis S, Hirsch N, Ip J. Anaesthesia, Intensive Care and Perioperative Medicine A-Z, 6th edition. Netherland: Elsevier, 2018.

Wong TY, Chong W, Yap Z, Farooqui S. The Ophthalmology Examinations Review, 3rd edition. London: World Scientific Publishing Company, 2019.

Bye L, Modi N, Stanford M. Basic Sciences for Ophthalmology (Oxford Specialty Training), 1st edition. Oxford: Oxford University Press, 2013.

Rowe FJ. Clinical Orthoptics, 3rd edition. Hoboken: Wiley-Blackwell, 2012.

American Academy of Ophthalmology. Basic and Clinical Science Course (13 volumes for 2021–2022 course). United States: American Academy of Ophthalmology, 2021.

Chapter 1

Exam Paper 1: Structured Practice Paper

Questions: SBAs

120 SBAs to be answered in 3 hours

For each question, please select the single best answer.

Anatomy

1. In the superior orbital fissure, which nerves pass outside the common tendinous ring?

    A   Lacrimal nerve, frontal nerve, abducens nerve
    B   Lacrimal nerve, frontal nerve, trochlear nerve
    C   Lacrimal nerve, nasociliary nerve, abducens nerve
    D   Lacrimal nerve, nasociliary nerve, frontal nerve

2. What is the horizontal diameter of the adult cornea?

    A   9.2 mm
    B   10.6 mm
    C   11.2 mm
    D   11.7 mm

3. Regarding the osteology of the skull, which of the following statements is false?

    A   Layers of compact bone are separated by a layer of spongy bone known as *diploë*
    B   Sutural ligament refers to the connective tissue between bones
    C   Sutures are mobile articulations
    D   The bones of the orbit include bones of the cranium and facial bones

4. Where does the frontal sinus drain into the nose?

    A   Inferior meatus
    B   Middle meatus

C Sphenoethmoidal recess
D Superior meatus

5. Which bones make up the medial wall of the orbit?
   A Ethmoid, lacrimal, maxilla
   B Ethmoid, nasal, lacrimal, maxilla
   C Sphenoid, ethmoid, lacrimal, maxilla
   D Sphenoid, nasal, palatine

6. Regarding the Meibomian glands, which of the following statements is correct?
   A Anterior blepharitis is characterised by Meibomian gland dysfunction
   B The Meibomian glands lie posterior to the grey line
   C There are approximately 150 Meibomian glands in the upper lid and 75 in the lower
   D They produce a mucinous secretion which is part of the tear film

7. Which of the following correctly describes the anatomy of the lacrimal gland?
   A Parasympathetic fibres reach the lacrimal gland via the pterygopalatine ganglion and zygomaticotemporal nerve
   B The lacrimal gland lies in the lacrimal fossa, formed by the lacrimal bone and maxilla
   C The lacrimal gland receives parasympathetic and sensory fibres, and has no sympathetic innervation
   D The parasympathetic innervation of the lacrimal gland is derived from the lacrimatory nucleus of the trigeminal nerve

8. Which one of the following statements accurately describes a property of extraocular muscle, when compared to skeletal muscle elsewhere in the body?
   A Muscle fibres of larger diameter are more peripherally placed in the muscle
   B The epimysium is generally thicker
   C The muscle fibres are more loosely packed, separated by connective tissue
   D The muscle spindles are shorter (<10 µm) and less numerous

9. Which one of the following structures does not pass through the foramen spinosum?
   A Meningeal branch of the facial nerve
   B Meningeal branch of the mandibular nerve
   C Middle meningeal artery
   D Middle meningeal vein

10. Which of the following nerves is not a branch of the facial nerve?
    A Buccal nerve
    B Frontal nerve

C   Mandibular nerve
D   Zygomatic nerve

11. Which of the following intracranial bleeds is typically a result of bleeding from the meningeal arteries?

    A   Extradural haematoma
    B   Intracerebral haemorrhage
    C   Subarachnoid haemorrhage
    D   Subdural haematoma

12. Schwalbe's line represents the termination of which corneal layer?

    A   Bowman's layer
    B   Corneal endothelium
    C   Corneal stroma
    D   Descemet's membrane

13. At which location is the lens capsule thinnest?

    A   Anterior pole
    B   Immediately anterior to the zonular insertion
    C   Immediately posterior to the zonular insertion
    D   Posterior pole

14. What is the site of attachment of the vitreous base?

    A   Fovea
    B   Optic disc and peripapillary region
    C   Peripheral retina and pars plana
    D   Posterior lens capsule

15. From outermost to innermost, which is the correct sequence of the layers of Bruch's membrane?

    A   Basement membrane of the choriocapillaris, outer collagenous layer, elastin layer, inner collagenous layer, basement membrane of the retinal pigment epithelium (RPE)
    B   Basement membrane of the choriocapillaris, outer collagenous layer, inner collagenous layer, elastin layer, basement membrane of the RPE
    C   Basement membrane of the RPE, outer collagenous layer, elastin layer, inner collagenous layer, basement membrane of the choriocapillaris
    D   Basement membrane of the RPE, outer collagenous layer, inner collagenous layer, elastin layer, basement membrane of the choriocapillaris

16. What is the point of insertion of the lateral canthal tendon?

    A   Eisler's tubercle
    B   Frontozygomatic suture

C Whitnall's tubercle
D Zygomaticomaxillary suture

17. Which of the following statements about the innervation of the iris is true?
    A Sensory innervation of the iris is derived from branches of the lacrimal nerve
    B The parasympathetic nerves to the iris synapse in the ciliary ganglion
    C The principal nerves to the dilator pupillae muscle originate in the Edinger–Westphal nucleus
    D The sphincter pupillae muscle is innervated by the long ciliary nerves

18. From posterior to anterior, what is the orientation of the optic canal?
    A Inferolateral
    B Inferomedial
    C Superolateral
    D Superomedial

19. Which statement about the ciliary body structure is false?
    A The blood supply to the ciliary body is via the anterior ciliary arteries and the long posterior ciliary arteries
    B The ciliary body has a greater nasal anteroposterior length than temporal anteroposterior length
    C The middle radial layer of the ciliary muscle is continuous with the corneoscleral meshwork
    D The outer longitudinal layer of the ciliary muscle attaches to the scleral spur

20. Which of the following statements about the blood supply to the iris is incorrect?
    A Iris capillaries are non-fenestrated
    B Most of the anastomoses between the major and minor arterial circles run through the anterior border layer
    C The major arterial circle of the iris receives blood from the anterior ciliary arteries
    D The minor arterial circle of the iris is at the level of the collarette

21. Into which vein do the lymphatics from the right side of the head and neck drain?
    A Right external jugular vein
    B Right internal jugular vein
    C Right lymphatic duct
    D Right subclavian vein

22. Regarding the microscopic structure of a blood vessel:
    A Fragmentation of the external elastic lamina is typically seen in giant cell arteritis
    B The internal elastic lamina is in the tunica intima

C   The tunica media is the main connective tissue layer of a blood vessel
D   Veins have relatively thicker tunica media than arteries

Biochemistry

23. Which one of the following substances is found in a lower concentration in aqueous compared with plasma?

    A   Ascorbate
    B   Glucose
    C   Lactate
    D   Sodium

24. Regarding collagen synthesis, which of the following statements is false?

    A   Collagen usually contains glycine at every third amino acid
    B   Glycosylation of collagen is vitamin C-dependent
    C   Post-translational modification occurs both in the endoplasmic reticulum and extracellularly
    D   The triple helix structure of collagen is linked by covalent S–S bonds

25. Regarding matrix metalloproteinases (MMPs), which of the following statements is correct?

    A   Endogenous inhibitors called TIMPs are present in normal tissues
    B   MMPs are magnesium-dependent proteins
    C   They are not required for normal tissue growth
    D   They are released mainly by B cells in acute inflammation

26. Regarding lens proteins, which of the following statements is false?

    A   Cytoplasmic interdigitations between lens fibres contain channels formed by MIP26 (aquaporin-0)
    B   Epithelial growth factor stimulates the differentiation of lens epithelial cells into lens fibres
    C   The differentiation of lens epithelial cells into lens fibres is characterised by a loss of organelles
    D   The genes encoding α-crystallin are found on chromosomes 21 and 11

27. Which of the following statements about glycosaminoglycans is false?

    A   Glycosaminoglycans are composed of long chains of repeating disaccharides
    B   Glycosaminoglycans are relatively inflexible molecules
    C   Glycosaminoglycans are strongly hydrophilic
    D   Glycosaminoglycans have a high positive charge

28. Which of the following best describes the actions of the corneal endothelial cell pump?

    A There is active transport of potassium into the aqueous
    B There is active transport of sodium into the aqueous
    C There is passive diffusion of sodium into the aqueous
    D There is passive diffusion of potassium into the corneal endothelial cell

29. Which one of the following vitamins is not lipid soluble?

    A Vitamin A
    B Vitamin C
    C Vitamin D
    D Vitamin K

30. Which of the following statements regarding pericytes is false?

    A Pericytes are contractile
    B Pericytes are embedded in the basement membrane of vessels
    C Pericyte coverage is highest in the choroid
    D Pericytes have an important role in the blood–brain barrier

31. Which of the following statements about vascular endothelial growth factor (VEGF) is false?

    A Aflibercept is an anti-VEGF monoclonal antibody
    B TNF-α upregulates VEGF synthesis
    C VEGF binds to receptors that act via intracellular tyrosine kinase
    D VEGF enhances permeability of vessels to macromolecules

32. Regarding photoreceptor segment renewal, which of the following statements is false?

    A Diurnal phagocytosis of rod outer segment tips occurs at first light
    B Melatonin synthesised by photoreceptors modulates rod disc shedding
    C Rod outer segments complete their renewal cycle every 21 days
    D Rod discs are phagocytosed in groups of approximately 200

Embryology, growth, and development

33. Which embryological cell population is the lens derived from?

    A Mesoderm
    B Neural crest-derived mesenchyme
    C Neural ectoderm
    D Surface ectoderm

34. In which quadrant are iris colobomas typically found?
    A Inferonasal
    B Inferotemporal
    C Superonasal
    D Superotemporal

35. Which pharyngeal arch gives rise to the orbicularis oculi muscle?
    A First pharyngeal arch
    B Second pharyngeal arch
    C Third pharyngeal arch
    D Fourth pharyngeal arch

36. At what gestational age does myelination of the optic nerve start?
    A Week 10
    B Week 16
    C Month 5
    D Month 7

37. Regarding the changes in the vitreous with age, which of the following is incorrect?
    A Hyaluronate pools and redistributes within the vitreous with age
    B Other than water, the main constituents of adult vitreous are type II collagen and hyaluronate
    C The vitreous is homogeneous during childhood, without visible collagen fibrils
    D The vitreous liquefies first in the periphery causing the posterior vitreous cortex to detach

Genetics

38. Which of the following conditions is not a result of autosomal trisomy?
    A Down syndrome
    B Edwards syndrome
    C Klinefelter syndrome
    D Patau syndrome

39. Regarding transcription, which of the following statements is true?
    A Introns are removed from the mRNA strand before it leaves the nucleus
    B RNA synthetase is the enzyme primarily responsible for creating the resultant RNA molecule

C The coding strand of DNA is copied to make a mirror RNA strand
D The resultant RNA molecule extends in a 3′ to 5′ direction

40. Which mode of inheritance is responsible for the transmission of Leber's hereditary optic neuropathy?

A Autosomal dominant
B Autosomal recessive
C Mitochondrial
D X-linked

41. Regarding mosaicism and chimerism, which of the following statements is false?

A All women are mosaics with respect to the X-chromosome genes
B Chimeras have genetically distinct cell populations arising from one zygote
C Individuals with cancer exhibit somatic mosaicism
D Infliximab is a murine–human chimeric monoclonal antibody

42. Regarding genetic linkage, which of the following statements is correct?

A Families undergoing linkage analysis need not express the phenotype of the allele in question
B Genetic loci on the same chromosome are normally expected to segregate together
C The aim of linkage analysis is to discover how often two loci are separated by mitotic recombination
D The probability of crossing over between two loci on the same chromosome is proportional to the distance between them

43. Which of the following statements regarding histones is false?

A Histone octamers are found at each nucleosome
B Histones can be dynamically modified to influence gene expression
C Histones contain a large quantity of lysine and arginine
D Histones have a high negative charge

44. Which of the following statements about mitochondrial genetics is false?

A DNA in mitochondria is double-stranded
B DNA polymerase β is the principal enzyme in mitochondrial DNA replication
C Mitochondrial chromosomes are circular
D Mitochondrial genomes contain genes for tRNA and rRNA

45. A 28-year-old patient with Reis–Buckler corneal dystrophy is pregnant. She already has a 10-year-old daughter who is unaffected. What is the risk of her child inheriting the condition?

A None
B 25%

    C   25% if her husband is a carrier
    D   50%

46. Regarding gene therapy, which of the following is not a vector used to transfer DNA into a cell?

    A   Adenoviruses
    B   Liposomes
    C   Retroviruses
    D   Ribozymes

Immunology

47. Which of the following is not a feature of the innate immune system?

    A   Complement cascade
    B   Mucosa-associated lymphoid tissue (MALT)
    C   NK cells
    D   Recognition of pathogen-associated molecular patterns (PAMPs)

48. Which of the following is not an antigen presenting cell?

    A   B cell
    B   Dendritic cell
    C   Monocyte
    D   T cell

49. Regarding major histocompatibility complex (MHC) class I molecules, which of the following statements is false?

    A   An example of an MHC class I molecule is HLA B27
    B   MHC class I molecules are present on every nucleated cell
    C   They present antigenic peptides on the surface of the cell
    D   Viral proteins presented with MHC class I molecules are recognised by CD4$^+$ T cells

Investigations and imaging

50. In which one of the following conditions would the electrooculogram (EOG) be normal?

    A   Advanced Stargardt macular dystrophy
    B   Best vitelliform macular dystrophy
    C   Optic neuritis
    D   Total retinal detachment

51. Which one of the following tissues appears bright on a T1-weighted MRI?
    A   Air
    B   Calcium
    C   Cerebrospinal fluid
    D   Fat

Microbiology

52. Regarding endophthalmitis, which of the following statements is false?
    A   *Bacillus cereus* is frequently implicated in chronic low-grade endophthalmitis
    B   Coagulase-negative staphylococci are frequently isolated in endophthalmitis following cataract surgery
    C   Exogenous endophthalmitis is more common than endogenous endophthalmitis
    D   *Pseudomonas* endophthalmitis causes severe tissue destruction by enzyme secretion

53. Which of the following is used for the culture of *Mycobacterium tuberculosis*?
    A   Löwenstein–Jensen medium
    B   MacConkey agar
    C   Sabouraud's agar
    D   Thayer–Martin medium

54. Which of the following antibiotics acts by inhibiting bacterial DNA-dependent RNA polymerase?
    A   Cefuroxime
    B   Chloramphenicol
    C   Rifampicin
    D   Vancomycin

55. What is the minimum time required for dry heat sterilisation at 160°C?
    A   30 minutes
    B   60 minutes
    C   120 minutes
    D   180 minutes

56. Which of the following statements about *Acanthamoeba* is true?
    A   *Acanthamoeba* keratitis is typically painless due to damage to corneal sensory nerve endings
    B   Chlorhexidine 0.02% and propamidine isetionate applied topically for a week will sterilise most *Acanthamoeba* infections

C   It can be grown on *Escherichia coli* nutrient-deficient agar
D   It is the most common cause of infective keratitis in contact lens wearers

57. By what mechanism does botulinum toxin A inhibit neurotransmission?
    A   Acetylcholine receptor antagonism
    B   Blockade of postsynaptic sodium channels
    C   Inhibition of acetylcholine exocytosis
    D   Intracellular blockade of acetylcholine production

58. Which of the following viruses does not typically cause keratitis?
    A   Adenovirus
    B   Cytomegalovirus
    C   Herpes simplex virus
    D   Varicella zoster virus

59. Which of the following is more typical of *Toxocara* than *Toxoplasma* infection?
    A   Infection via ingestion of animal faeces
    B   Leucocoria
    C   Vitritis
    D   White chorioretinal lesions

60. Regarding *Haemophilus influenzae*:
    A   It is a cause of orbital cellulitis
    B   It is a Gram positive anaerobe
    C   Encapsulated serotypes are less virulent
    D   Vaccination covers most virulent serotypes

Optics

61. What is the magnification of a loupe of power +16 dioptres?
    A   × 4
    B   × 8
    C   × 32
    D   × 64

62. An object lies outside the centre of curvature of a concave mirror. How is the image formed by the mirror best described?
    A   Real, inverted, diminished
    B   Real, inverted, enlarged
    C   Virtual, erect, diminished
    D   Virtual, erect, enlarged

63. A crown glass prism in air has an apical angle of 4°. What will the angle of deviation be in the position of minimum deviation?

   A 2°
   B 4°
   C 8°
   D 16°

64. How is the image formed by a convex lens of an object located within the first focal point best described?

   A Erect, real, inside the second focal point, diminished
   B Erect, virtual, further from lens than object, magnified
   C Inverted, real, outside the second focal point, magnified
   D Inverted, virtual, at infinity, diminished

65. What is the maximum amplitude of accommodation of an emmetropic patient with a near point of 20 cm?

   A 2 dioptres
   B 5 dioptres
   C 8 dioptres
   D 10 dioptres

66. What are the units of illuminance (luminous flux incident at a surface per unit area)?

   A Candela
   B Candela/m^2
   C Lux
   D Watt/m^2

67. Regarding Jackson's cross cylinder:

   A It is equivalent to two superimposed cylindrical lenses with axes at 45° to each other
   B The cylinder in the cross cylinder has twice the power of the sphere
   C The handle is traditionally in line with the axis of the negative cylinder
   D When checking the power of the trial cylinder during refraction, the cross cylinder's handle is held in line with the axis of the trial cylinder

68. Which of the following statements regarding the Prentice position is incorrect?

   A Glass prisms are traditionally held in the Prentice position
   B The angle of incidence equals the angle of emergence
   C The deviation of light is greater in the Prentice position than in the position of minimum deviation
   D The incident ray is normal to one surface of the prism

69. Regarding the reflection of light:
    A A glass door appears transparent because no reflection of light occurs
    B At a curved surface, the angle of reflection is equal to half the angle of incidence
    C The incident ray, reflected ray and the reflecting surface are all in the same plane
    D When a plane mirror is rotated by 45°, light reflected on the centre of rotation is deviated by 90°

70. Which of the following best describes the image formed by reflection of an object at a plane mirror?
    A Real, erect, laterally inverted
    B Real, as far behind the surface as the object is in front of it, magnified
    C Virtual, erect, diminished
    D Virtual, erect, laterally inverted

71. Regarding the refraction of light, which of the following statements is incorrect?
    A The angle of refraction and the normal to the refracting surface both lie in the same plane
    B The refractive index of the human crystalline lens is 1.386–1.406
    C When entering an optically less dense medium, light is deviated away from the normal
    D When light passes from air to Crown glass, the angles of incidence (i) and refraction (r) are related as follows:
    $$1.52 = \frac{\cos i}{\cos r}$$

72. What is the spherical equivalent of –3.50/+1.50 axis 70°?
    A –2.00 DS
    B –2.00/–1.50 axis 160°
    C –2.75 DS
    D –5.00 DS/+1.50 DC axis 160°

73. During cataract surgery a complication occurs and the decision is made to place the intraocular lens (IOL) in the sulcus. A 23.5 dioptre IOL had been planned for placement in the capsular bag. Which of the following lens powers is most appropriate for placement in the sulcus?
    A 21.5 dioptre
    B 22.5 dioptre
    C 24.5 dioptre
    D 25.5 dioptre

74. Which of the following statements about the Maddox rod is false?
    A A distant spot target is viewed with a Maddox rod over one eye only
    B It is composed of parallel high-powered convex cylindrical lenses
    C The glass of the Maddox rod is clear to eliminate chromatic aberration
    D The line seen through the Maddox rod lies at 90° to the axis of the rod

75. Which one of the following is not a test of stereoacuity?
    A Cardiff cards
    B Frisby
    C Titmus
    D Worth 4-dot

76. Comparing direct and indirect ophthalmoscopy, which of the following statements is false?
    A A patient's refractive error has a greater effect on indirect ophthalmoscopy
    B Direct ophthalmoscopy gives greater magnification
    C Indirect ophthalmoscopy gives an image that is inverted vertically and horizontally
    D The field of view is greater with an indirect ophthalmoscope

77. In simple hypermetropic astigmatism:
    A Both focal lines are behind the retina
    B Both focal lines are in front of the retina
    C One focal line is on the retina whilst the other is behind it
    D The focal lines are straddling the retina

78. A patient's prescription is +2.00 DS/−1.00 DC axis 180°. What is the toric transposition of this to the base curve −4 D?

    A $\dfrac{+1.00 \text{ DS}}{-5.00 \text{ DC axis } 180° \,/\, +1.00 \text{ DC axis } 90°}$

    B $\dfrac{+1.00 \text{ DS}}{+1.00 \text{ DC axis } 90° \,/\, -5.00 \text{ DC axis } 180°}$

    C $\dfrac{+6.00 \text{ DS}}{-4.00 \text{ DC axis } 90° \,/\, -5.00 \text{ DC axis } 180°}$

    D $\dfrac{+6.00 \text{ DS}}{-4.00 \text{ DC axis } 180° \,/\, -1.00 \text{ DC axis } 90°}$

79. Which of the following indirect ophthalmoscopy lenses gives the widest field of view?
    A 15 D
    B 20 D

C 28 D
D 30 D

80. Which of the following best describes the image produced by a Galilean telescope?

    A Virtual, erect, magnified, at infinity
    B Virtual, erect, magnified, at the sum of the focal lengths of the objective and eyepiece lens
    C Virtual, inverted, magnified, at infinity
    D Virtual, inverted, magnified, at the sum of the focal lengths of the objective and eyepiece lens

81. Regarding optical radiation, which of the following statements is false?

    A Light emitted through fluorescence typically has a longer wavelength than the excitation light that triggers it
    B Shorter wavelengths undergo increased scatter
    C The energy of a photon is directly proportional to its wavelength
    D The wavelength of light decreases as it enters a transparent material from a vacuum

82. Which one of the following statements about interference is correct?

    A Destructive interference is used in anti-reflection coatings
    B Laser light generates less interference than conventional light sources
    C The corneal stroma uses constructive interference in maintaining clarity
    D Two waves of equal amplitude out of phase by one cycle will cancel each other out

83. Regarding the prevalence of myopia (of at least −0.5 dioptres):

    A It is high in white Europeans compared to other ethnicities
    B It is lower in adults than in young children
    C Myopia tends to decrease with nuclear sclerosis of the lens
    D Time spent outdoors as a child is a protective factor against myopia

Pathology

84. Which of the following tumours is not associated with neurofibromatosis?

    A Acoustic neuroma
    B Meningioma
    C Phaeochromocytoma
    D Renal cell carcinoma

85. In which of the following conditions are Dalen–Fuchs nodules seen?
   A   Best disease
   B   Coats disease
   C   Retinitis pigmentosa
   D   Sympathetic ophthalmia

86. What percentage of uveal tract melanomas arise from the ciliary body?
   A   12%
   B   24%
   C   36%
   D   48%

87. Which of the following statements about myasthenia gravis is false?
   A   An ice pack applied over the affected muscles for 5 minutes characteristically causes a temporary improvement in symptoms
   B   Autoantibodies are produced which target skeletal muscle acetylcholine receptors
   C   In Cogan's lid twitch, the upper lid overshoots when returning to the primary position from downgaze and there is a subsequent compensatory downward 'twitch'
   D   There is characteristic muscle wasting, often involving facial and extraocular muscles

88. Which of the following terms is used to refer to an increase in the number of cells in a tissue?
   A   Dysplasia
   B   Hyperplasia
   C   Hypertrophy
   D   Metaplasia

89. Which of the following statements regarding amyloid is false?
   A   Amyloid appears as a homogenous blue material on haematoxylin and eosin (H&E) staining
   B   In lattice dystrophy, amyloid deposits occur in the corneal stroma
   C   Systemic amyloidosis is more common than localised amyloidosis
   D   When stained with Congo red, amyloid shows 'apple' green birefringence when exposed to polarised light

90. Where in the retina are hard exudates found?
   A   Between the photoreceptors and the RPE
   B   Ganglion cell layer
   C   Nerve fibre layer
   D   Outer plexiform layer

91. Which of the following does not describe typical corneal arcus?

    A   Age-related
    B   Fatty degeneration
    C   Stromal lipid deposition
    D   Unilateral

92. Regarding retinal detachment:

    A   Accumulation of subretinal fluid occurs in all types of retinal detachment
    B   Rhegmatogenous detachment is commonly inflammatory or vascular
    C   The outer blood–retinal barrier is intact in serous retinal detachment
    D   The retinal pigment epithelium is usually separated from the choriocapillaris

93. Regarding proliferative vitreoretinopathy, which of the following is least correct?

    A   Contraction of fibrous membranes leads to retinal detachment
    B   Fibrosis and collagen production contribute to retinal membranes
    C   Raised intraocular pressure is common, due to inflammation
    D   RPE cell migration into the vitreous is characteristic

94. A 30-year-old man sustains a full-thickness corneal laceration. Which of these is not part of the wound healing process?

    A   Fibrin plug formation and stromal oedema
    B   Regeneration of the epithelium and Bowman's layer
    C   Replacement of damaged stroma by scar tissue
    D   Transformation of aqueous-derived leucocytes into fibroblasts

Pharmacology

95. Which of the following is not an effect of botulinum toxin A?

    A   Brief blockade of synaptic transmission
    B   Cleavage of SNARE proteins required for fusion of neurosecretory vesicles with the plasma membrane
    C   Inhibition of the exocytosis of acetylcholine at the neuromuscular junction
    D   Parasympathetic and motor nerve paralysis

96. Regarding pharmacokinetics, which of the following statements is true?

    A   Eye drops absorbed in the systemic circulation via the nasopharyngeal mucosa undergo first-pass metabolism
    B   First-order kinetics are nonlinear
    C   Highly protein-bound drugs tend to distribute easily into tissues
    D   Lipid-soluble drugs can pass the blood–retinal barrier

97. Which of the following is not a side effect of ciclosporin?

    A   Bone marrow suppression
    B   Gingival hypertrophy
    C   Hirsutism
    D   Nephrotoxicity

98. A patient with a known Pancoast tumour of the lung is referred to the eye clinic with anisocoria. This is more pronounced in darker conditions with the right pupil failing to dilate. Which of the following agents is likely to succeed in dilating both pupils?

    A   Cocaine 4%
    B   Hydroxyamphetamine 1%
    C   Pilocarpine 1%
    D   None of the above

99. What is the mechanism of action of brimonidine?

    A α_2 agonist
    B β antagonist
    C   Carbonic anhydrase inhibitor
    D   Prostaglandin analogue

100. Which of the following is not a side effect of acetazolamide?

    A   Hyperkalaemia
    B   Metabolic acidosis
    C   Paraesthesia
    D   Renal stones

101. Regarding eicosanoids, which of the following statements is true?

    A   Eicosanoids are derived from cyclooxygenase
    B   Nonsteroidal anti-inflammatory drugs (NSAIDs) inhibit the biological actions of eicosanoids on their target tissue
    C   NSAIDs reduce eicosanoid synthesis via inhibition of lipoxygenase
    D   Thromboxane A_2 causes vasoconstriction

102. Which of the following benzodiazepines has the shortest half-life?

    A   Diazepam
    B   Lorazepam
    C   Midazolam
    D   Temazepam

Physiology

103. Which of the following results from activation of histamine H_1 receptors?
    A Decreased intracellular calcium concentration
    B Increased gastric acid production
    C Increased vascular permeability
    D Mast cell degranulation

104. Which of the following statements regarding colour vision is true?
    A As illuminance decreases retinal sensitivity to red light increases
    B Chromaticity is an objective measure of colour quality
    C Green cones have maximum spectral sensitivity at 590 nm
    D Hues are perceived as more red at high illuminance

105. Which of the following statements about dark adaptation is true?
    A Full dark adaptation takes approximately two hours
    B In a dark adapted subject, a greater intensity of light is required to elicit a rod response than a cone response
    C Increased cone sensitivity accounts for the early component of the dark adaptation curve
    D Light adaptation is much slower than dark adaptation

106. Which of the following statements regarding potassium is incorrect?
    A Daily dietary potassium requirements are approximately 1 mmol/kg/day
    B Insulin promotes the movement of potassium from the intracellular to the extracellular compartment
    C Potassium is reabsorbed by the proximal convoluted tubule and secreted by the distal convoluted tubule of the nephron
    D The concentration of potassium in intracellular fluid is 135–150 mmol/L

107. Regarding the cardiac cycle, which of the following statements is false?
    A Atrial depolarisation corresponds to the p-wave on an ECG
    B Atrial contraction is responsible for 80% of ventricular filling
    C Mitral valve closure precedes tricuspid valve closure
    D Passive filling of the ventricles is rapid in early diastole

108. Regarding the hypothalamic–pituitary axis, which of the following statements is incorrect?
    A Gigantism is caused by over-secretion of growth hormone
    B Somatostatin promotes the release of growth hormone from the anterior pituitary

C The hypothalamic hormones are sometimes referred to as 'factors'
D The release of anterior pituitary hormones is pulsatile

109. Which of the following processes is not thought to contribute to aqueous humour production?

   A Active secretion
   B Oncotic pressure
   C Passive diffusion
   D Ultrafiltration

110. Neurons from the optic radiations terminate in which layer of the primary visual cortex?

   A 1
   B 2
   C 3
   D 4

111. Which of the following statements about the organisation of the primary visual cortex is false?

   A Cells from layer 6 provide 'feed-forward' innervation to the lateral geniculate nucleus
   B Cells in layer 5 project principally to the secondary visual cortex
   C Fibres representing the superior retina terminate in the superior lip of the calcarine sulcus
   D Ocular dominance columns each respond to a single eye, alternating between columns

112. Which of the following functions is thought to be directed by the suprachiasmatic nucleus?

   A Auditory/visual integration
   B Circadian rhythm
   C Co-ordination of head and eye movements
   D Pupillary light reflex

113. Which glycosaminoglycan is thought to be most important in maintaining corneal clarity?

   A Chondroitin sulphate
   B Dermatan sulphate
   C Heparan sulphate
   D Keratan sulphate

114. Which of the following statements about action potentials in neurons is false?
    A Action potentials are classically generated by a sudden influx of Na⁺ ions into the neuron
    B Action potentials are triggered at the initial segment of the axon
    C Between action potentials, neurons maintain a negatively charged resting membrane potential
    D The magnitude of an action potential determines the quantity of neurotransmitter released

115. Which of the following eye movements is disconjugate?
    A Saccadic eye movements
    B Smooth pursuit movements
    C Vergence movements
    D Vestibulo-ocular movements

116. Which of the following is not a correct pair of yoked muscles?
    A Left inferior oblique and right superior rectus
    B Left medial rectus and right lateral rectus
    C Right inferior oblique and left superior oblique
    D Right superior oblique and left inferior rectus

117. Which of the following is not a part of the accommodation response?
    A Ciliary muscle relaxation
    B Convergence
    C Increase in lens curvature
    D Miosis

118. Regarding hearing, which of the following statements is incorrect?
    A Depolarisation of hair cells in the cochlea occurs due to the influx of sodium
    B Higher frequencies are detected by hair cells near the base of the cochlea
    C Sound is audible to humans between 20 and 20,000 Hz
    D Sound is converted by the organ of Corti into action potentials in the auditory nerve

Statistics and evidence-based medicine

119. A new test is being validated against the definitive gold standard test. 50 patients are tested positive by the gold standard test. Of these patients, 35 tested positive using the new test. A further five patients tested positive with the new test, but were found to be negative using the gold standard test. What is the sensitivity of the new test?

A 50%
B 60%
C 70%
D 80%

120. In a clinical study, what is the correct definition of a type II error?
    A Failing to reject the null hypothesis when it is false
    B Failing to reject the null hypothesis when it is true
    C Rejecting the null hypothesis when it is false
    D Rejecting the null hypothesis when it is true

Questions: CRQs

12 CRQs to be answered in 2 hours

Anatomy

1.

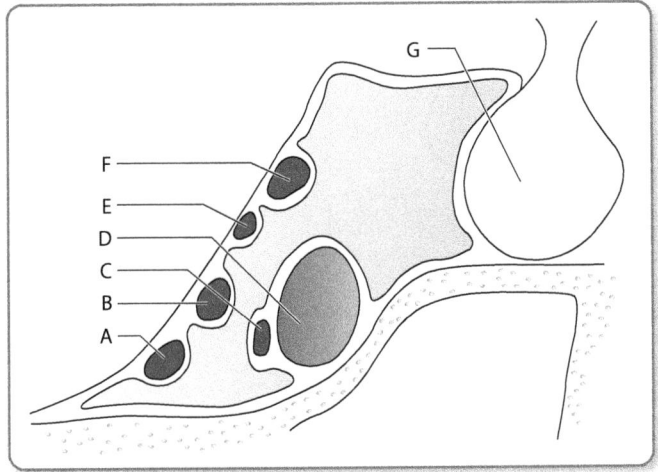

(a) Identify the structures labelled A to G on the diagram showing a coronal section through the body of the sphenoid bone. (7 marks)
(b) Name two conditions affecting the venous system which typically affect this area of the body. (2 marks)
(c) Which cranial nerve is most commonly impaired in conditions affecting this area? (1 mark)

Biochemistry and cell biology

2. Below is a diagram of a sympathetic synapse at the dilator pupillae muscle.

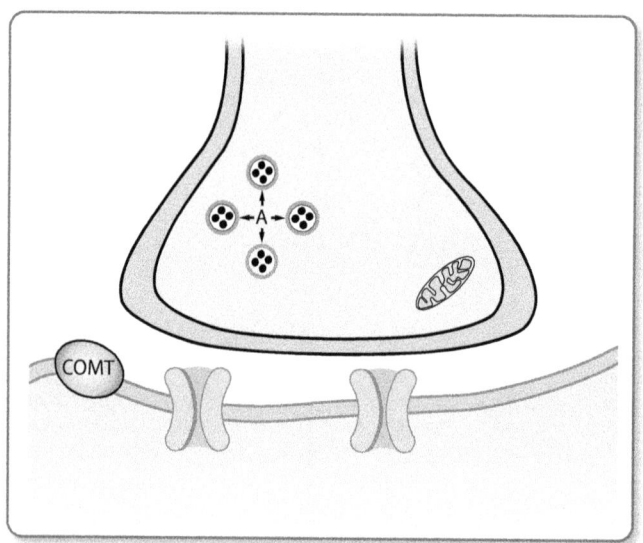

(a) What are the microstructures labelled 'A'? (1 mark)
(b) What is the principal neurotransmitter at this synaptic terminal? (1 mark)
(c) Which amino acid is this neurotransmitter synthesised from? (1 mark)
(d) Name two other neurotransmitters that are synthesised from this amino acid. (2 marks)
(e) What is the cellular process used to release neurotransmitters? (1 mark)
(f) What are the two types of receptor found at synapses, as defined by their mechanism of signal transduction, and which type is responsible for transmission at this synapse? (3 marks)
(g) What is the principal neurotransmitter at the synapse in the superior cervical ganglion? (1 mark)

Genetics

3. A family comes to the ocular genetics clinic to discuss their condition. The proband is 32 years old. Ocular examination shows marked bilateral iris hypoplasia, nystagmus and reduced vision. She is registered partially sighted, works as a lawyer and is pregnant with her second child.

The proband's father (aged 65) is affected, and has bilateral absence of the iris, keratopathy, bilateral pseudophakia, nystagmus, and is registered blind. Her mother (64) is unaffected. The proband has two unaffected siblings (male, 36; female, 29). Her youngest male sibling died in a car accident aged 23, but was also unaffected by the condition.

The proband has an affected daughter (14 months) with bilateral iris hypoplasia and nystagmus. The proband's husband has no eye conditions or relevant family history.

(a) Draw a pedigree (family tree) for this family. (5 marks)
(b) What is the likely mode of inheritance? (1 mark)
(c) What is the risk of her unborn child being affected? Please state whether the risk is affected by the sex of the child. (2 marks)
(d) State the most likely diagnosis. (1 mark)
(e) Which gene is most commonly responsible for this condition? (1 mark)

Investigations and imaging

4.

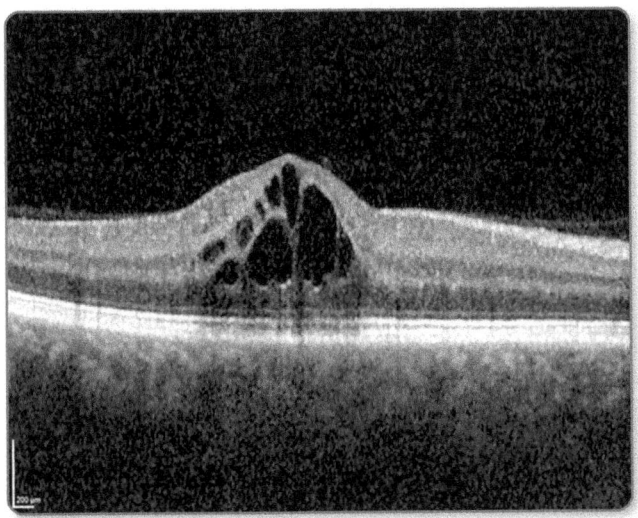

(a) What is the name of this investigation? (1 mark)
(b) How is the image produced? (3 marks)
(c) Describe two limitations of this investigation. (2 marks)
(d) What is the principal abnormality in this scan? (1 marks)
(e) Give two possible diagnoses which could cause the above abnormality. (2 marks)
(f) What further retinal investigation could you order if the diagnosis was unclear? (1 mark)

5. The biometry below relates to one patient who is attending for consideration of cataract surgery (first eye).

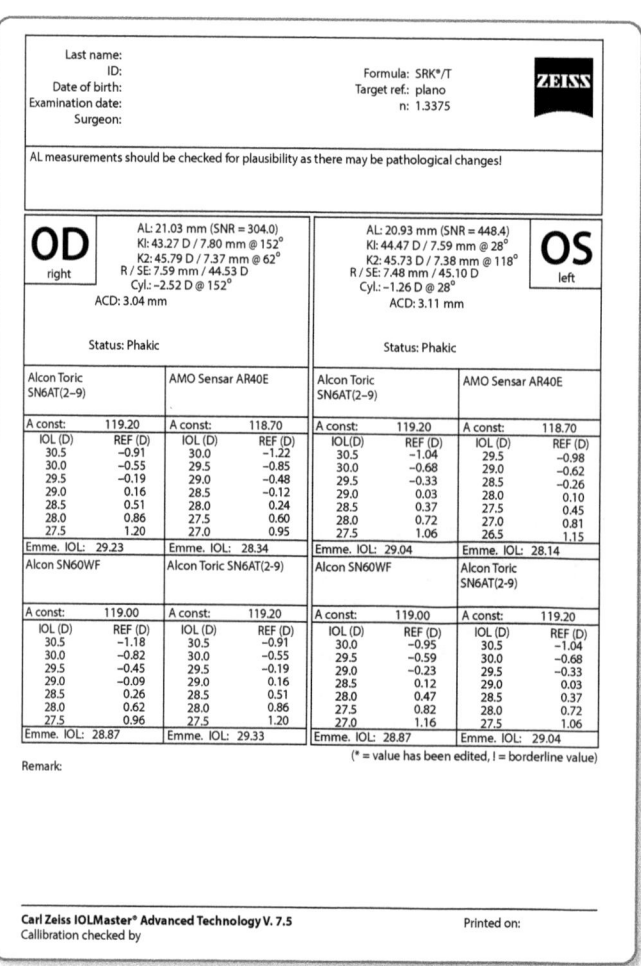

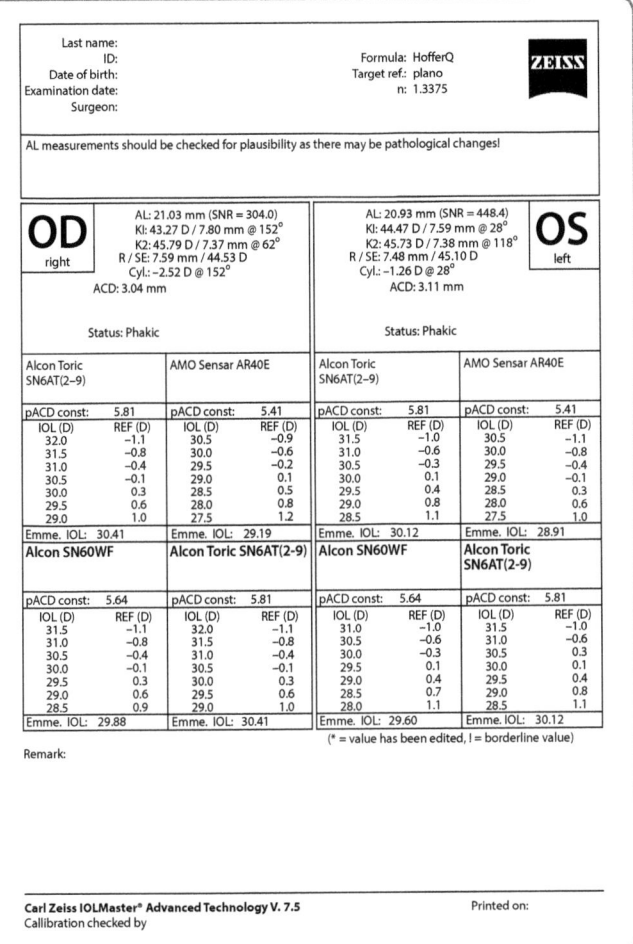

(a) Which of these two formulae is likely to be more accurate for the left eye, and which measurement allows you to determine this? (2 marks)
(b) Which two biometric measurements of the eye are used in both the SRK/T and Hoffer Q formulas? (2 marks)
(c) Which parameter is typically different when measured with contact ultrasound as opposed to immersion or optical biometry, and what causes the difference? (2 marks)
(d) What is the principal disadvantage of optical biometry? (1 mark)
(e) Which two positions could you make your incision in the right eye if you wanted to reduce astigmatism? (2 marks)
(f) Refer to the SRK/T biometry. If the SN60WF IOL's A-constant is 119.0, and a further lens type has a predicted outcome of −0.09 for a 28.5 dioptre IOL in the right eye, what is the A-constant of this new IOL? (1 mark)

6. Below are images from two different investigations in the same eye of the same patient.

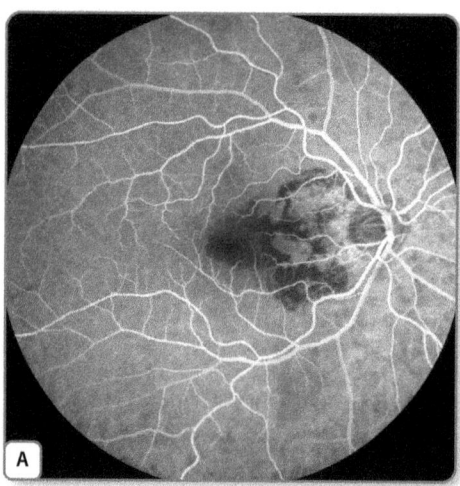
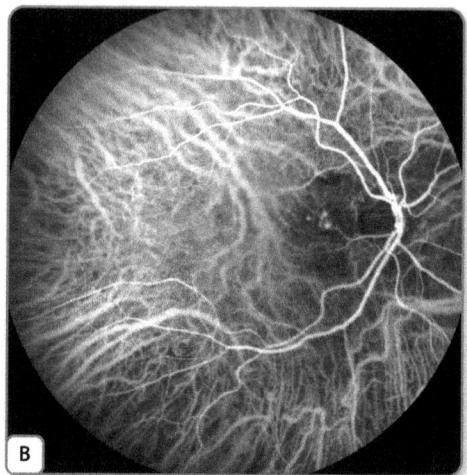

(a) What is the investigation labelled B above? (1 mark)

(b) In which part of the electromagnetic spectrum are the excitation source and fluorescence for investigation B? (2 marks)

(c) Give two reasons why the choroidal circulation cannot be well visualised with fluorescein angiography. (2 marks)

(d) In addition to providing better imaging of the choroidal circulation, give three further advantages of investigation B over fluorescein angiography. (3 marks)

(e) Why is the leakage of dye slower in investigation B than in fluorescein angiography? (1 mark)

(f) What is the mechanism of excretion of the dye used in investigation B? (1 mark)

7. Below are two axial CT images of the same patient from the same study.

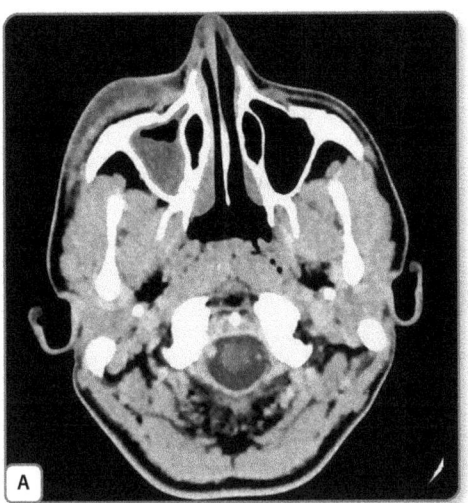
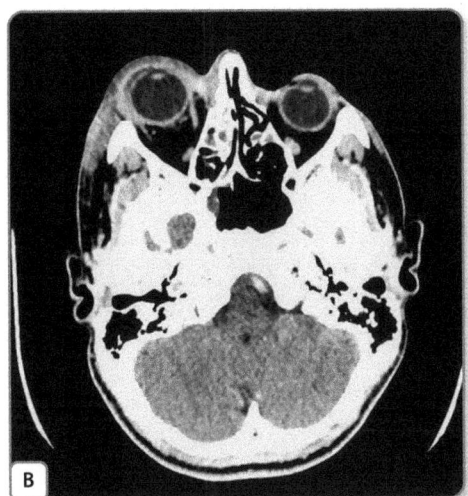

(a) Describe how the images in a CT scan are obtained. (2 marks)
(b) What are the two principal abnormalities in image A? (2 marks)
(c) What further clinically significant abnormality can be seen in image B? (1 mark)
(d) What is the most likely diagnosis? (1 mark)
(e) What pupil abnormality would you look for and what is its significance? (2 marks)
(f) Name two possible intracranial complications of this condition. (2 marks)

Microbiology

8. A 36-year-old male recently returned from Bangladesh is seen in the eye casualty department with a corneal ulcer which developed following an abrasion. Microscopy of the scrape is shown below:

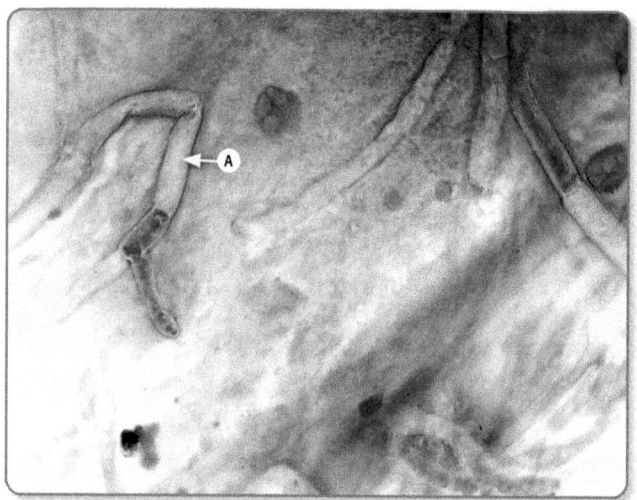

   (a) What can be seen at A? (1 mark)
   (b) What culture medium would be appropriate? (1 mark)
   (c) What is the principal limitation of culture in this case? (1 mark)
   (d) Name two specialist stains that could be used on this specimen in combination with a fluorescent microscope. (2 marks)
   (e) Suggest two possible genera given this patient's history and corneal scrape. (2 marks)
   (f) Name three risk factors for this form of keratitis. (3 marks)

Optics

9. Right eye +1.50 DS/+1.50 DC axis 75°   Left eye −1.50 DS/+0.75 DC axis 95°
   (a) Express the above refractions in negative cylinder form. (2 marks)
   (b) What is the spherical equivalent of the right eye? (1 mark)
   (c) The patient is pseudophakic in the left eye but phakic in the right. She normally wears glasses. Name three options to address this lady's anisometropia. (3 marks)

(d) If this patient develops increasing nucleosclerosis in her right eye, the anisometropia may decrease. Why is this? (1 mark)
(e) Describe two methods of reducing this lady's astigmatism during her right cataract surgery. (2 marks)
(f) When making a corneal incision, how will moving the incision site further from the limbus affect induced corneal astigmatism? (1 mark)

10.
(a) Draw a diagram of Gullstrand's schematic eye, clearly labelling the first and second focal points; first and second principal points, and first and second nodal points. (6 marks)
(b) In which part of the eye is the nodal point located in the reduced schematic eye? (1 mark)
(c) Why does the cornea account for a greater proportion of the total refractive power of the eye than the lens, when the refractive index of the lens is greater than that of the cornea? (3 marks)

11. Two patients attend the paediatric eye clinic. Orthoptic examination and cycloplegic refraction reveal the following:

Patient 1, aged 6
Visual acuity: 6/6 right eye, 6/7.5 left eye (Snellen acuity)
Interpupillary distance: 55 mm
Prism cover test (PCT): Near (33 cm or 3 D): +8 prism dioptres (Δ) esophoria
Distance: $-4\,\Delta$ exophoria
Cycloplegic refraction: +2.00 DS right eye, +2.50 DS left eye

Patient 2, aged 4
Visual acuity: 0.200 right eye, 0.150 left eye (logMAR acuity using crowded Kay Pictures)
PCT: esotropia (without glasses) measuring 30 Δ for near and distance
Accommodative convergence/accommodation (AC/A) ratio: 6:1
Cycloplegic refraction: +5.00 DS in each eye

(a) What is meant by the term 'AC/A ratio'? (2 marks)
(b) What is the normal range for the AC/A ratio? (1 mark)
(c) Calculate the AC/A ratio for patient 1, using the heterophoria method; show your working. (4 marks)
(d) Patient 2 is prescribed the full hypermetropic glasses correction. What effect will this have on the esotropia? Please quantify this and show your working. (3 marks)

12.

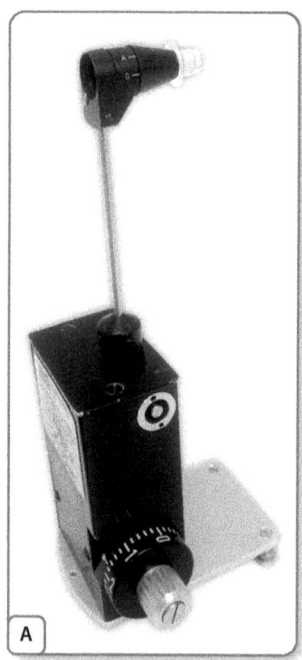
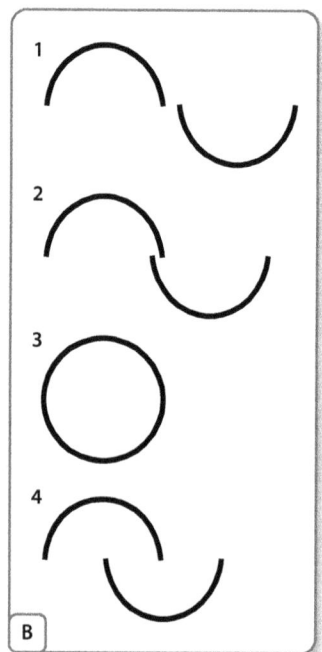

(a) What instrument is shown in part A? (1 mark)
(b) Explain how prisms are used in taking a measurement. (2 marks)
(c) With the aid of a diagram, explain the principle behind and forces involved in taking a measurement. (4 marks)
(d) In part B, which diagram shows that the force applied is too low? (1 mark)
(e) Please give two factors which may lead to an inaccurate measurement. (1 mark)
(f) How would interpretation of the test be affected in a patient with a corneal pachymetry reading of 620 μm? (1 mark)

Answers: SBAs

Anatomy

1. **B Lacrimal nerve, frontal nerve, trochlear nerve**

   The nerves passing outside the common tendinous ring are the lacrimal, frontal and trochlear nerves. The superior and inferior divisions of the oculomotor nerve, the nasociliary nerve and the abducens nerve pass within the common tendinous ring. There are several mnemonics based on the first letters of each nerve: LFT SNIA.

2. **D 11.7**

   The diameter of the adult cornea is 11.7 mm horizontally and 10.6 mm vertically. At birth, the horizontal diameter is approximately 10 mm, with the adult size reached by 2 years of age.

3. **C Sutures are mobile articulations**

   The skull comprises separate bones which are joined by connective tissue known as sutural ligament. Sutures are immobile, rigid articulations. A tiny amount of flex is permitted at the sutures to aid skull elasticity, but not enough to classify the articulations as mobile. *Diploë* is the name of the spongy bone that separates tables of compact bone. The bones of the orbit include some bones of the cranium (frontal, sphenoid, and ethmoid) and some of the facial bones (zygomatic, maxilla, palatine, and lacrimal).

4. **B Middle meatus**

   The paranasal sinuses all drain into the nose. Their opening sites into the nasal cavity are summarised in **Table 1.1**.

Table 1.1 Opening sites of the paranasal sinuses	
Sinus	Site of opening into nose
Frontal	Middle meatus
Maxillary	
Ethmoidal (anterior and middle groups)	
Ethmoidal (posterior group)	Superior meatus
Sphenoidal	Sphenoethmoidal recess or superior meatus

5. **C Sphenoid, ethmoid, lacrimal, maxilla**

   The bones of the medial wall of the orbit are, from posterior to anterior: the body of the sphenoid, the orbital plate of the ethmoid, the lacrimal bone and the maxilla. The orbital plate of the ethmoid, or lamina papyracea, forms the paper-thin separation between the orbit and the ethmoid sinuses. The lacrimal bone and maxilla form the lacrimal fossa, which houses the lacrimal sac.

Table 1.2 below summarises the bones of the four orbital walls. Note that the sphenoid forms part of all except the orbital floor. Whereas the roof and lateral wall are simpler with only two bony structures, some find the medial wall and floor easier to remember by their acronyms, SELM and ZyMP.

Table 1.2 Bones of the four orbital walls	
Orbital wall	**Constituent bones**
Medial wall	Sphenoid (body), ethmoid, lacrimal, maxilla
Floor	Zygomatic, maxilla, palatine
Lateral wall	Zygomatic, sphenoid (greater wing)
Roof	Frontal, sphenoid (lesser wing)

6. B The Meibomian glands lie posterior to the grey line

The Meibomian glands, also known as tarsal glands, are embedded in the tarsal plates. Their openings, approximately 30–40 in the upper lid and 20–30 in the lower lid, are visible at the slit lamp posterior to both the lash line and the grey line. They are modified sebaceous glands which produce an oily substance that forms part of the precorneal tear film. This lipid layer reduces the rate of evaporation of tears. This explains why patients who are prone to blocked Meibomian glands, which is often called Meibomian gland dysfunction or posterior blepharitis, may experience dry eye symptoms. Anterior blepharitis involves crusting/debris and inflammation around the lash line, and the two often coexist.

A chalazion is a lipogranulomatous inflammatory cyst resulting from a blocked Meibomian gland.

7. A Parasympathetic fibres reach the lacrimal gland via the pterygopalatine ganglion and zygomaticotemporal nerve

The lacrimal gland lies in the superolateral orbit and consists of an orbital and a palpebral portion. It is important to read the question properly and avoid confusion with the lacrimal sac, which lies in the lacrimal fossa and is involved in drainage rather than production of tears.

The innervation of the lacrimal gland is autonomic and sensory, as follows:

- Parasympathetic supply, from the lacrimatory nucleus of the facial (seventh) nerve. These fibres travel via the nervus intermedius to the pterygopalatine ganglion, then via the maxillary nerve to its zygomatic and zygomaticotemporal branches, and finally via the lacrimal nerve to the gland. (Note that the maxillary and lacrimal nerves themselves are branches of the

trigeminal nerve, but these parasympathetic fibres from the facial nerve nucleus are carried along with them).
- Sympathetic supply, from the superior cervical ganglion. These fibres travel in the nerve plexus surrounding the internal carotid artery, then via the deep petrosal nerve to the maxillary nerve. From there, the course to the lacrimal gland is as for the parasympathetic fibres above.
- Sensory supply, from the lacrimal nerve, which is a branch of the trigeminal nerve (V1).

8. C The muscle fibres are more loosely packed, separated by connective tissue

There are important differences between extraocular muscles and normal skeletal muscle found elsewhere in the body. The connective tissue of the extraocular muscles, including the epimysium (a sheath surrounding the whole muscle) is generally thin and delicate by comparison. The muscle fibres are more loosely packed, with the larger diameter (10–40 μm) fibres occupying the centre and the smaller fibres (5–15 μm) placed peripherally in the muscle. Extraocular muscle also has many specialised sensory and proprioceptive endings, including long muscle spindles almost 1 mm in length, which provide feedback about muscle activity to the central nervous system. Lastly, extraocular muscle is more vascular than normal skeletal muscle.

9. A Meningeal branch of the facial nerve

The facial nerve does not have a meningeal branch. The other three structures pass through the foramen spinosum, which connects the middle cranial fossa with the infratemporal fossa.

10. B Frontal nerve

The frontal nerve is derived from the ophthalmic (V1) branch of the trigeminal nerve. There is a useful mnemonic for the branches of the facial nerve that has a number of variations. One publishable version is Two Zebras Bit My Coccyx:

T – temporal nerve

Z – zygomatic nerve

B – buccal nerve

M – mandibular nerve

C – cervical nerve

11. A Extradural haematoma

The meningeal arteries, and in particular the middle meningeal artery and its dural branches, are vulnerable to injury from cranial trauma. This is particularly true in the temporal region, where the pterion is prone to fracture. As these vessels are extradural they typically result in an extradural haematoma (the pressure of arterial bleeding is required to create a plane between bone and dura).

12. D Descemet's membrane

Schwalbe's line marks the termination of Descemet's membrane. It is often visible clinically using gonioscopy and is visible as a smooth zone with scanning electron microscopy.

13. D Posterior pole

The lens capsule is thinnest at the posterior pole (2–3 µm). The anterior pole is 9–14 µm and in the peri-zonular region the capsule is 17–28 µm thick. This is an important consideration during cataract surgery, particularly when approaching soft lens matter adherent to the posterior pole.

14. C Peripheral retina and pars plana

The vitreous base is a three-dimensional band that extends approximately 2 mm either side of the ora serrata and is usually attached to the peripheral retina and pars plana. It is firmly adherent, and clean dissection during vitrectomy surgery is very hard to achieve. It is extremely important that an adequate visualisation of the peripheral retina is achieved in cases of posterior vitreous detachment, as any resultant tears are likely to lie in this region.

15. A Basement membrane of the choriocapillaris, outer collagenous layer, elastin layer, inner collagenous layer, basement membrane of the retinal pigment epithelium (RPE)

Bruch's membrane is composed of five layers: the basement membrane of the choriocapillaris, an outer collagenous layer, an elastin layer, an inner collagenous layer and the basement membrane of the RPE.

16. C Whitnall's tubercle

The lateral canthal tendon inserts into Whitnall's tubercle, which is a small prominence of bone lying just inside the lateral orbital rim. Eisler's fat pad lies immediately anterior to the lateral canthal tendon, deep to the orbital septum, and is a useful surgical landmark for identifying Whitnall's tubercle.

17. B The parasympathetic nerves to the iris synapse in the ciliary ganglion

The parasympathetic nerves supplying the iris originate in the Edinger–Westphal nucleus and synapse in the ciliary ganglion. Their postganglionic fibres travel via the short ciliary nerves and supply the sphincter pupillae muscle. The dilator pupillae is predominantly innervated by unmyelinated sympathetic fibres originating in the superior cervical sympathetic ganglion. The sensory innervation of the iris is via both the long and short ciliary nerves, which derive from the nasociliary nerve (and ultimately V1).

Answers: SBAs

18. **A Inferolateral**

    From posterior to anterior the optic canal runs slightly inferiorly and around 36° laterally through the sphenoid. It is narrowest at the orbital opening and widens posteriorly. It connects the middle cranial fossa and the orbital apex.

19. **B The ciliary body has a greater nasal anteroposterior length than temporal anteroposterior length**

    The ciliary body has a greater anteroposterior length temporally than nasally, and is generally at its longest inferotemporally. It varies with the size of the globe, measuring 5.6–6.3 mm temporally and 4.6–5.2 mm nasally. The other statements are true. The third (innermost) muscle layer is composed of circular fibres. The ciliary body stroma lies between the ciliary muscle and the ciliary epithelium.

20. **B Most of the anastomoses between the major and minor arterial circles run through the anterior border layer**

    The anterior border layer of the iris normally contains very few blood vessels, and significant vascularisation suggests ischaemic insult. There are extensive anastamoses between the major and minor arterial circles which run predominantly through the iris stroma in a radial manner. Iris capillaries are non-fenestrated with tight junctions and pericytes, contributing to the blood–ocular barrier. The major arterial circle (which is often incomplete) derives its blood supply from the anterior ciliary arteries (which travel anteriorly with the extraocular muscles before piercing the sclera) and the long posterior ciliary arteries (which pierce the sclera near the optic nerve and run anteriorly between the sclera and choroid to the ciliary body). The minor arterial circle of the iris is at the level of the collarette, and is also often incomplete. From here vessels continue inwards to the pupillary border.

21. **D Right subclavian vein**

    The lymphatic ducts from the right side of the head and neck, and the right arm, drain into the right subclavian vein. The final common lymphatic duct before entering the venous system is the right lymphatic duct.

    The thoracic duct collects lymph from the rest of the body and drains into the left subclavian vein.

    The blood from the subclavian veins returns to the heart via the brachiocephalic veins and superior vena cava.

22. **B The internal elastic lamina is in the tunica intima**

    The three principal layers (tunica) of blood vessels, from the lumen outwards, are as follows:

    1. Intima
    2. Media
    3. Adventitia

The tunica intima contains the endothelium supported by the internal elastic lamina. The latter is typically fragmented in giant cell arteritis.

The tunica media is the main muscular layer of the vessel. It contains smooth muscle cells, and varying amounts of elastic fibres (principally in medium to large arteries).

The tunica adventitia (sometimes called tunica externa) is the main connective tissue layer, and in arteries this contains the external elastic lamina.

Veins have a thinner tunica media, larger lumen, and contain proportionally less muscle and less elastic tissue than arteries.

Biochemistry

23. B Glucose

Compared to plasma, aqueous contains:

- Higher levels of lactate and ascorbate;
- Similar concentrations of sodium, potassium, and magnesium;
- Slightly lower levels of bicarbonate;
- Lower levels of glucose and calcium (about half that of plasma), and much lower levels of albumin

24. B Glycosylation of collagen is vitamin C-dependent

The steps of collagen synthesis are summarised in **Table 1.3**. The end result is an insoluble, extracellular glycoprotein.

Table 1.3 Steps of collagen synthesis

Stage of collagen synthesis	Further details
Transcription	DNA → RNA
Translation	RNA → peptide formation The basic amino acid sequence is repeating triplets $(Glycine\text{-}X\text{-}Y)_n$ where X is often proline, Y is often hydroxyproline Polypeptides (primary structure) twist into a left-handed helix (secondary structure; ≠ α-helix)
Post-translational modification (endoplasmic reticulum)	Vitamin C-dependent hydroxylation of the Y-position amino acid Glycosylation Triple helix formation (tertiary structure) linked by covalent S–S bonds
Excretion from the cell	Cleavage of terminal peptide chains, making it insoluble
Extracellular modification	Lysine oxidation Formation of crosslinks

25. A Endogenous inhibitors called TIMPs are present in normal tissues

Matrix metalloproteinases (MMPs) are zinc and calcium-dependent endopeptidases which act as an enzyme cascade to degrade extracellular matrix. They can potentially degrade all types of extracellular matrix, and include collagenases and gelatinases. MMPs are released by neutrophils during the acute inflammatory response (they mediate cell and tissue damage, along with free radicals from the respiratory burst), and also by cells in normal tissues for growth, maintenance, repair, and remodelling. For example, when stimulated by growth factors, one of the responses of a cell is to release MMPs to degrade the surrounding extracellular matrix to create space for the increase in cell numbers. They are kept in check by endogenous tissue inhibitors of MMPs (TIMPs).

26. B Epithelial growth factor stimulates the differentiation of lens epithelial cells into lens fibres

One-third of the weight of the lens is protein, and 90% of the lens protein is composed of crystallins. Secondary lens fibres are formed from the anterior lens epithelium. Fibroblast growth factor (FGF) is one of the principal factors that stimulate the differentiation of anterior lens epithelial cells into lens fibres. This change is characterised by elongation, withdrawal from the cell cycle, expression of large amounts of crystallins, and eventually the loss of organelles and the nucleus.

Lens fibres are densely packed, with cytoplasmic interdigitations and intercellular, gap junction-like channels formed by MIP26 (main intrinsic polypeptide 26), which was subsequently recognised as an aquaporin and named aquaporin-0 (AqP0).

The genes encoding the two types of α-crystallin (known as αA and αB) are found on chromosomes 21 and 11, respectively.

27. D Glycosaminoglycans have a high positive charge

Glycosaminoglycans have a high negative charge. They are polysaccharides composed of long chains of repeating disaccharides. Unlike proteins, they are inflexible. As highly charged molecules they are strongly hydrophilic, and form a gel that is resistant to compression. With the exception of hyaluronan they may be found as sulphated molecules, and may be attached to a protein, forming a proteoglycan. The functions of these proteoglycans are extremely diverse.

28. B There is active transport of sodium into the aqueous

The corneal endothelial cell pump moves sodium and bicarbonate from the stroma to the aqueous by active transport. This is mediated by a sodium/potassium-dependent ATPase and a bicarbonate-dependent ATPase, and is facilitated by co-transporters. Potassium and chloride move to the aqueous predominantly by passive diffusion.

29. **B Vitamin C**

    Vitamins A, D, E, and K are lipid soluble, whereas vitamins B and C are water soluble. Lipid soluble vitamins can be stored in the liver and adipose tissue, whereas water soluble vitamins must be consumed more regularly. Patients with either reduced lipid intake or reduced lipid absorption may develop deficiencies of lipid soluble vitamins, as they are normally absorbed in chylomicrons.

30. **C Pericyte coverage is highest in the choroid**

    Pericyte coverage is highest in the retinal vessels, with a relative frequency of 1:1 pericytes to endothelial cells. This may be because of the meticulous metabolic demands of the retina, and the requirement to maintain the blood–retinal barrier.

    Conversely the vessels of the choroid have a much less dense coverage of pericytes, facilitating exchange of metabolites. Pericytes are contractile cells embedded in the basement membrane of vessels, to which they contribute. They are involved in a number of regulatory functions, communicating with the endothelial cells by paracrine signalling and direct contact. They play a key role in maintaining the blood–brain barrier, where they regulate permeability. They may also have a role in controlling cerebral blood flow.

31. **A Aflibercept is an anti-VEGF monoclonal antibody**

    Aflibercept is a fusion protein acting as a decoy receptor molecule for VEGF (it contains binding domains from type 1 and type 2 VEGF receptors). Bevacizumab is a monoclonal antibody to VEGF, and ranibizumab is a monoclonal antibody fragment from the same mouse antibody. VEGF synthesis is upregulated by a large number of metabolic and growth factors including TNF-α, TNF-β, IL-1α, IL-6, prostaglandin E2, epidermal growth factor, fibroblast growth factor, insulin-like growth factor-1, keratinocyte growth factor and platelet-derived growth factor. All three identified VEGF receptors act via intracellular tyrosine kinase. In addition to promoting the division and survival of vascular endothelial cells, VEGF promotes vascular dilatation and increased permeability to macromolecules. It also has functions in regulating gene expression, cell migration, and nitric oxide production.

32. **C Rod outer segments complete their renewal cycle every 21 days**

    About 10% of the rod outer segment is phagocytosed daily, and it takes 9–10 days for the renewal cycle to be complete. Melatonin is synthesised by photoreceptors in conditions of darkness and suppresses dopamine production. Conversely, local dopamine production increases during conditions of light and suppresses melatonin production. These mechanisms are involved in modulating the circadian rhythm of photoreceptor renewal, with rod disc shedding and phagocytosis occurring at first light. Cone outer segments are predominantly shed at the onset of darkness. Rod discs are phagocytosed in groups of approximately 200. It is hard to measure cone segment phagocytosis experimentally.

Embryology, growth, and development

33. D Surface ectoderm

The lens originates from a thickening of surface ectoderm called the lens placode, which invaginates to form the lens vesicle. By day 36 this separates from the remaining surface ectoderm. The surrounding basal lamina will later form the lens capsule.

34. A Inferonasal

Colobomas are a result of failed or incomplete closure of the embryonic optic fissure, and are thus found inferonasally. The fissure is important for allowing the hyaloid artery to be incorporated into the developing globe.

35. B Second pharyngeal arch

The orbicularis oculi muscle, like all muscles of facial expression, is derived from the second pharyngeal arch. The muscular contributions of the pharyngeal arches are summarised in **Table 1.4**.

Table 1.4 Muscular contributions of the pharyngeal arches	
Pharyngeal arch	Muscular contributions
1	Muscles of mastication (masseter, pterygoids, and temporalis); mylohyoid; tensor tympani; tensor veli palatini; anterior belly of digastric
2	Muscles of facial expression (surrounding the eye these include orbicularis oculi; corrugator supercilii; depressor supercilii; procerus and occipitofrontalis); stylohyoid; stapedius; posterior belly of digastric
3	Stylopharyngeus
4	Pharyngeal constrictors, levator veli palatini, cricothyroid
5	None (regresses during embryogenesis)
6	Intrinsic muscles of the larynx except cricothyroid

36. D Month 7

Axons grow from developing retinal ganglion cells, changing course at the optic disc and growing towards the optic stalk and brain.

Optic nerve fibres are present from week 6 to 7. Myelination starts from the optic chiasm in month 7 of gestational development, but continues after birth. It is complete by 1 to 3 months of age in a full term baby.

37. D The vitreous liquefies first in the periphery causing the posterior vitreous cortex to detach

In childhood, type II collagen and hyaluronate gradually increase in concentration in the vitreous, which is homogeneous without visible fibrils. In adulthood, fibrils become visible due to the dissociation of hyaluronate and collagen, and aggregation of the latter.

The central vitreous is the first to liquefy. The vitreous reduces in size, and liquefied vitreous (from pooling of hyaluronate) escapes into the subhyaloid space, leading to posterior vitreous detachment.

Genetics

38. C Klinefelter syndrome

Klinefelter syndrome is caused by an additional X chromosome, rather than an additional autosomal chromosome (trisomy 21 for Down syndrome; trisomy 18 for Edwards syndrome; trisomy 13 for Patau syndrome).

39. A Introns are removed from the mRNA strand before it leaves the nucleus

Introns are removed from the mRNA strand and the remaining exons are spliced together before the molecule leaves the nucleus. The enzyme primarily responsible for creating the RNA molecule during transcription is RNA polymerase. This binds to the template strand of DNA which is copied to make a mirror RNA strand. The coding strand of DNA is the opposite strand of DNA which therefore corresponds directly to the resultant RNA sequence. RNA polymerase reads the DNA strand in a 3' to 5' direction, and therefore extends the resultant RNA strand in a 5' to 3' direction.

40. C Mitochondrial

As only the mother's mitochondria are passed on, the offspring of an affected male will not inherit the condition. Another mitochondrial-inherited condition with ophthalmological manifestations is Kearns–Sayre syndrome.

41. B Chimeras have genetically distinct cell populations arising from one zygote

The terms mosaic and chimera apply to an organism composed of cells of two or more genotypes. In mosaicism, the cells all arise from the same zygote. In chimerism, the cells arise from two or more zygotes.

Somatic mosaicism occurs naturally in all women due to the process of X-inactivation (lyonisation), where one X-chromosome of their somatic cells is randomly inactivated. It occurs by day 12 of embryonic development, with all descendants of that cell having the same functional X-chromosome (either maternal or paternal). This can give rise to patchy expression of mutant X-linked genes. Somatic mosaicism also occurs in cancer cells, with mutations in the proliferating tumour cell line that are not found in normal cells.

The term chimera can be applied more broadly in science, for example to proteins (*Chimera* is the name of a mythical ancient Greek creature that was part lion, part goat and part serpent). Some monoclonal antibodies are chimeric fusion proteins. For example, murine B cells producing antibodies against a desired target can be genetically engineered to introduce human constant domains, reducing the chance of immune rejection. Monoclonal antibodies whose name ends *–ximab* fall into this category (e.g. infliximab), whereas 'fully humanised' monoclonal antibodies end in *–zumab*.

42. D The probability of crossing over between two loci on the same chromosome is proportional to the distance between them

If two genetic loci are on different chromosomes, they will segregate independently when gametes are formed by meiosis. The converse is not true: if they are on the same chromosome, they do not always segregate together due to the fact that crossing over (recombination) occurs between non-sister chromatids during prophase I of meiosis.

Linkage analysis is a statistical approach to identifying the chromosomal location of a disease gene by analysing how often two loci are separated by meiotic recombination (not mitotic). The probability of crossing over between two genetic loci on the same chromosome is proportional to the distance between them. This can be used to map the chromosomal location of unknown genetic variants, using a co-inherited genetic marker whose chromosomal location is known.

Families undergoing linkage analysis need to express a clear phenotype. By establishing genetic markers of known loci with the affected and non-affected phenotypes, linkage analysis can provide information about the genetic status of family members at risk of the condition. Highly polymorphic genetic loci are the most informative for linkage analysis, as they are heterozygous in a large proportion of the population.

Linkage is particularly useful in cases where the exact mutation cannot be identified in a family, so direct DNA analysis is not possible.

43. D Histones have a high negative charge

Histones have a high positive charge, allowing them to associate with DNA which has a negative charge. Lysine and arginine are positively charged (basic) amino acids, and are found in large numbers in histones.

Histones form octamers which act as the core of each nucleosome. DNA is wound round the histone core, and the resultant nucleosomes are assembled into chromatin.

Histones can be dynamically modified by a number of post-translational modifications, occurring predominantly on the accessible histone 'tails'. These modifications alter histone–DNA binding and influence gene expression.

44. B DNA polymerase β is the principal enzyme in mitochondrial DNA replication

DNA polymerase γ is the principal enzyme in mitochondrial DNA replication. The alpha subunit of this enzyme is encoded by the *POLG* gene on chromosome 15. Mutations in *POLG* can lead to a number of mitochondrial diseases including chronic progressive external ophthalmoplegia (both autosomal dominant and autosomal recessive forms) and Alpers' syndrome. The circular double-stranded DNA of mitochondria encodes 22 tRNAs, 2 rRNAs, and a number of polypeptides required for oxidative phosphorylation.

45. D 50%

Reis–Buckler corneal dystrophy has an autosomal dominant inheritance pattern and so the risk to offspring is 50%. Apart from macular corneal dystrophy and congenital hereditary endothelial dystrophy, which are autosomal recessive, and Lisch epithelial corneal dystrophy, which is X-linked dominant, it is generally safe to assume that a corneal dystrophy is autosomal dominant.

Reis–Buckler is characterised by granular deposits in the epithelial basement membrane, Bowman's layer and anterior stroma. These stain red with Masson's trichrome. It manifests clinically as recurrent corneal erosion and corneal opacification which may require corneal grafting.

46. D Ribozymes

Gene therapy aims to treat a genetic condition by replacing the abnormal gene with a healthy one or by manipulating its expression.

Vectors are used to insert the DNA into the chromosome of the cell, and these can be divided into viral and non-viral vectors. Viral vectors exploit the normal viral transfection/transduction abilities to deliver the desired gene, and include adenoviruses, retroviruses, adeno-associated viruses, and herpes simplex viruses. Non-viral vectors include liposomes and naked DNA in the form of plasmids. More recently, gene editing technologies such as CRISPR-Cas9 are facilitating more precise editing of DNA.

Ribozymes are also a tool in gene therapy but they are not vectors: they can be used to downregulate or repair genes involved in pathogenesis via their cleaving and splicing properties.

Immunology

47. B Mucosa-associated lymphoid tissue (MALT)

The main components of the innate immune system are as follows:

1. Physical: physicochemical barriers, e.g. eyelids, tears, skin

2. Chemical:
   i. molecules present in body fluids, e.g. complement, antiproteases, C-reactive protein, lysozyme
   ii. molecules released by cells when needed, such as cytokines (e.g. interferons and TNF-α). These molecules are also released by antigen-specific cells as part of the acquired immune system
3. Cells: phagocytic and cytotoxic cells, e.g. macrophages, neutrophils, and NK cells

MALT, which contains lymphocytes, is a component of the acquired immune system. The principal characteristics of the innate immune system, compared to the acquired, are that it is more rapid and less specific. Whilst the acquired immune system generates receptors specific to a particular epitope, the innate immune system is either non-specific in its response, or broadly specific. An example of the latter is the group of receptors on cells such as phagocytes which recognise pathogen-associated molecular patterns (PAMPs). PAMPs are well-conserved molecular structures that are often shared by related pathogens, such as the flagellin of bacterial flagella.

There is a lot of interaction between the innate and acquired immune systems; for example IgM antibodies are potent activators of the complement system.

48. D T cell

Antigen presenting cells (APCs) include: monocytes, macrophages, dendritic cells, some B cells, and activated endothelial cells. They constitutively express MHC class II molecules.

T cells are not APCs. The main function of APCs is to allow T cells to recognise antigens.

49. D Viral proteins presented with MHC class I molecules are recognised by CD4$^+$ T cells

T cells do not respond to peptide antigen that is free in solution. For a T cell to recognise an antigen, the antigen must be presented on the cell surface in association with major histocompatibility complex (MHC) molecules.

MHC class I molecules are present on every nucleated cell, whereas MHC class II molecules are only expressed by antigen presenting cells (APCs). HLA-B27 is an example of an MHC class I molecule.

Intracellular antigens such as viral proteins form a complex with MHC class I molecules and are presented to CD8$^+$ T cells. By contrast, extracellular antigen (which has been digested by the APC into short peptides) is presented with MHC class II molecules for recognition by CD4$^+$ T cells.

Investigations and imaging

50. C Optic neuritis

From an electrical point of view, the eye functions as a dipole. The electro-oculogram (EOG) measures the resting electrical potential between the retinal pigment epithelium (electrically negative) and cornea (positive). It is tested under both dark- and light-adapted conditions, and requires a cooperative patient who can make horizontal eye movements.

It is essentially a test of the function of the outer retina and retinal pigment epithelium (RPE), so is abnormal in conditions with a generalised disruption of the RPE-photoreceptor interface or in conditions with generalised RPE disease.

The EOG is normal in optic nerve disease. Two classic examples of diseases in which the EOG is abnormal are Best vitelliform macular dystrophy and acute zonal occult outer retinopathy (AZOOR).

51. D Fat

MRI scanning has a number of different imaging sequences, and in particular it is important to know the distinction between T1-weighted and T2-weighted images. Key differences in tissue appearance are summarised in **Table 1.5**.

Table 1.5 Tissue appearances on MRI: T1 versus T2

Tissue	T1-weighted MRI	T2-weighted MRI
Air	Black	Black
Dense bone	Black	Black
Calcium	Black	Black
Low protein fluid (e.g. cerebrospinal fluid)	Dark	Bright
White matter	Grey	Dark
Grey matter	Grey	Grey
Acute blood	Grey	Dark
Subacute blood	Bright	Bright
Fat	Bright	Moderately bright
High-protein fluid (e.g. highly concentrated mucus)	Bright	Dark

Microbiology

52. A *Bacillus cereus* is frequently implicated in chronic low-grade endophthalmitis

Bacillus cereus causes a rapidly progressing endophthalmitis which is devastating to the ocular tissues, causing advanced tissue damage within 12–24 hours.

Coagulase-negative staphylococci have been isolated in nearly 70% of cases of endophthalmitis following cataract surgery in several studies.

Endogenous endophthalmitis is rare, accounting for fewer than 10% of all cases of endophthalmitis.

Pseudomonas species produce a number of enzymes which promote tissue destruction and limit the efficacy of some antimicrobials.

53. A Löwenstein–Jensen medium

Löwenstein–Jensen medium is optimised to culture *Mycobacterium tuberculosis*, while inhibiting the growth of other bacteria. This is necessary due to the slow doubling time of *M. tuberculosis* (15–20 hours) and resultant long incubation. Sabouraud's agar is used to culture fungi and filamentous bacteria. Thayer–Martin medium is useful for isolating *Neisseria* species. MacConkey agar is used to grow cultures of Gram negative bacteria, and to determine whether they are lactose fermenting.

54. C Rifampicin

Rifampicin inhibits bacterial DNA-dependent RNA polymerase, blocking the synthesis of bacterial RNA. Chloramphenicol binds to the 50s subunit of the bacterial ribosome, inhibiting bacterial protein synthesis. Vancomycin and cefuroxime inhibit bacterial cell wall synthesis.

55. D 180 minutes

Dry heat sterilisation takes considerably longer than moist heat sterilisation. Exposure time is inversely related to the temperature of exposure. Minimum sterilisation times for dry and moist heat are shown in **Table 1.6** (as per World Health Organization guidelines).

Table 1.6 Minimum sterilisation times for dry and moist heat

Temperature (°C)	Minimum sterilisation time (min)
Moist Heat	
121–124	15
126–129	10
134–138	5
Dry heat	
160	180
170	60
180	30

56. **C It can be grown on *Escherichia coli* nutrient-deficient agar**

    Acanthamoeba may be grown on *E. coli* nutrient-deficient agar from samples including corneal scrapes and contact lens cases. Acanthamoeba keratitis is characterised by pain in excess of what might be expected from clinical findings. While Acanthamoeba keratitis is more common in contact lens wearers than the general population it is still far less common than bacterial keratitis. Acanthamoeba exists both as trophozoites and as cysts. Trophozoites are relatively sensitive to treatment, but cysts can take many weeks to eradicate.

57. **C Inhibition of acetylcholine exocytosis**

    Botulinum toxin A is a protein produced by *Clostridium botulinum*, a Gram positive bacteria. It is internalised by cholinergic nerve terminals and inhibits the exocytosis of acetylcholine.

58. **B Cytomegalovirus**

    Cytomegalovirus (CMV) typically causes uveitis (anterior and/or posterior). CMV retinitis is an important cause of visual loss in immunocompromised individuals. Whilst CMV can rarely cause keratitis, in the form of corneal endotheliitis, keratitis is a much more common presentation of the other three viruses listed.

    Viral keratitis is often associated with inflammation in other ocular structures. For example adenovirus causes keratoconjunctivitis, and herpes zoster (varicella zoster virus) causes keratouveitis. Herpes simplex is a common cause of recurrent keratitis, which may affect the corneal epithelium (e.g. dendritic ulceration), stroma or endothelium, giving rise to different clinical pictures.

59. **B Leucocoria**

    Toxocara infection (toxocariasis) is a nematodal infection that typically affects children. It causes posterior uveitis and is part of the differential diagnosis for leucocoria. Both *Toxocara* and *Toxoplasma* can be transmitted to humans via ingestion of animal faeces. *Toxocara canis* ova are shed in dog faeces; *Toxocara cati* ova and *Toxoplasma gondii* cysts are shed in cat faeces. Both *Toxocara* and *Toxoplasma* cause white chorioretinal lesions and, in some cases, vitritis. Infection may be asymptomatic.

60. **A It is a cause of orbital cellulitis**

    Haemophilus influenzae is an aerobic, Gram negative bacillus. The descriptor coccobacillus is often applied, as the rods are very small and can give the appearance of cocci. *Haemophilus influenzae* is best cultured on chocolate agar with added X and V factors. The organism was believed to be responsible for influenza, before it was established to be a viral infection.

    It is a common cause of respiratory tract infections and sinusitis, the latter becoming orbital cellulitis if spread through the orbital wall occurs.

    The virulence of the serotype is related to the capsule, with encapsulated serotypes being more virulent and invasive. Encapsulated strains are classified on the basis of capsular antigens into serotypes a–f. Vaccination is only routinely available against *Haemophilus influenzae* type b, a serotype associated with meningitis particularly in young children. The Hib vaccine, as it is known, is part of the routine vaccination schedule in the UK.

Optics

61. **A ×4**

    The nominal magnification power of a loupe is given by the equation:

    $$M = \frac{F}{4}$$

    where M is the magnification and F is the power of the lens in dioptres. This is derived using the standard near point of an adult eye, accepted as 25 cm (1/4 m).

62. **A Real, inverted, diminished**

    Objects outside the centre of curvature of a concave mirror will produce an image that is real, inverted and diminished, lying between the centre of curvature and the principal focus. It is always worth drawing the ray diagram for these questions. One ray runs from the top of the object parallel to the principal axis, and is reflected through the principal focus. The other runs from the top of the object through the centre of curvature and will therefore hit the mirror at 90° to the surface and be reflected along the same path. The image is formed where these two rays intersect. This is demonstrated in **Figure 1.1**, where O represents the object position, I represents the image position, C represents the centre of curvature, and F represents the principal focus (located half-way between C and the mirror).

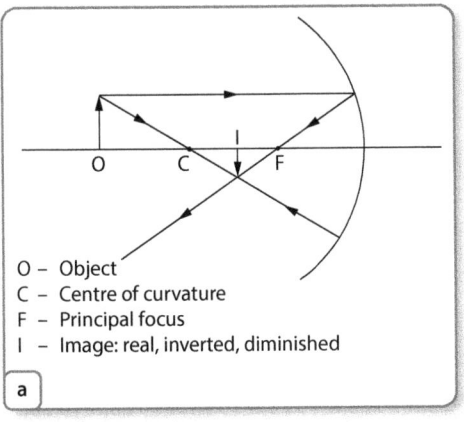

a

O – Object
C – Centre of curvature
F – Principal focus
I – Image: real, inverted, diminished

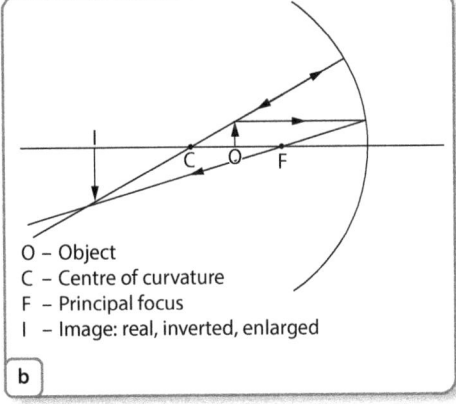

b

O – Object
C – Centre of curvature
F – Principal focus
I – Image: real, inverted, enlarged

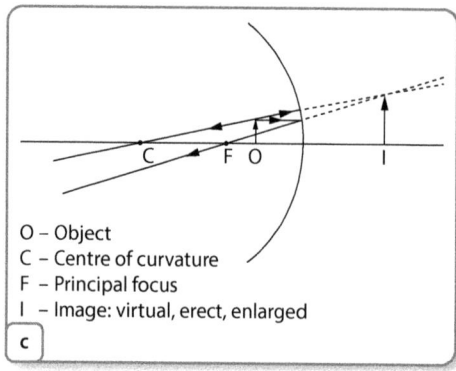
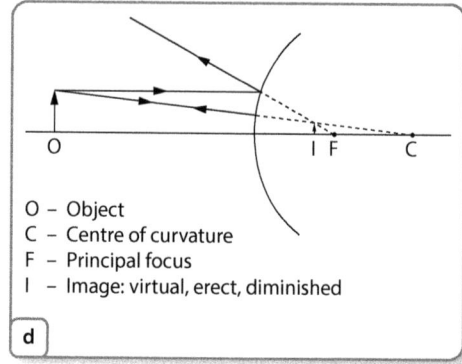

Figure 1.1 Reflection at curved mirrors.

63. **A 2°**

    The angle of deviation in a prism in the position of minimum deviation is defined by the formula:

    $$D = (n - 1)\alpha$$

    where D is the angle of deviation, n is the refractive index and α is the apical angle.

    Crown glass has a refractive index of 1.52, so for any crown glass prism in air:

    $$D = (1.52 - 1)\alpha$$

    $$\approx \frac{\alpha}{2}$$

64. **B Erect, virtual, further from lens than object, magnified**

    An object located within the first focal point of a convex lens will produce an image that is erect, virtual, further from the lens than the object and magnified. It is always worth drawing the ray diagram for these questions. One ray runs from the top of the object parallel to the principal axis, and is refracted through the second principal focus (note that in the case of concave lenses it is a virtual ray that passes through the second principal focus). The other runs from the top of the object through the principal point at the centre of the lens, and continues undeviated. The image is formed where these two rays intersect. This is demonstrated in **Figure 1.2**, where O represents the object position, I represents the image position, F_1 represents the first principal focus and F_2 represents the second principal focus.

Figure 1.2 Refraction by convex and concave lenses.

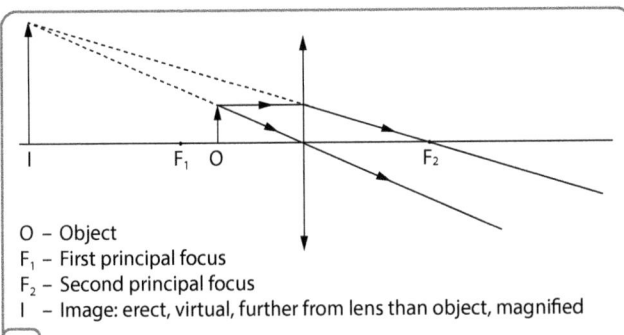

O – Object
F_1 – First principal focus
F_2 – Second principal focus
I – Image: erect, virtual, further from lens than object, magnified

a

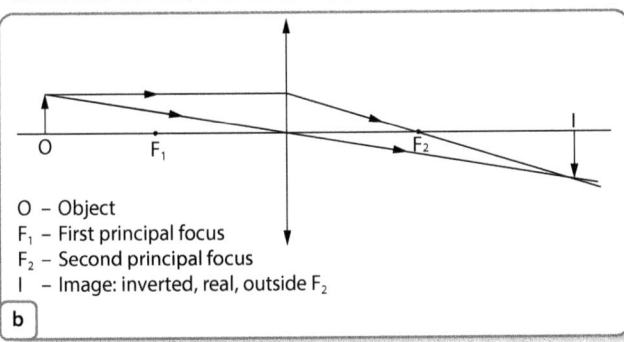

O – Object
F_1 – First principal focus
F_2 – Second principal focus
I – Image: inverted, real, outside F_2

b

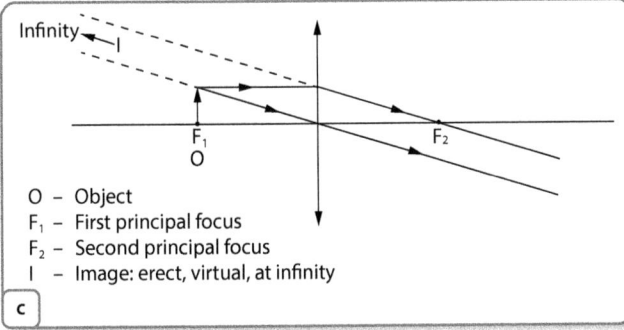

O – Object
F_1 – First principal focus
F_2 – Second principal focus
I – Image: erect, virtual, at infinity

c

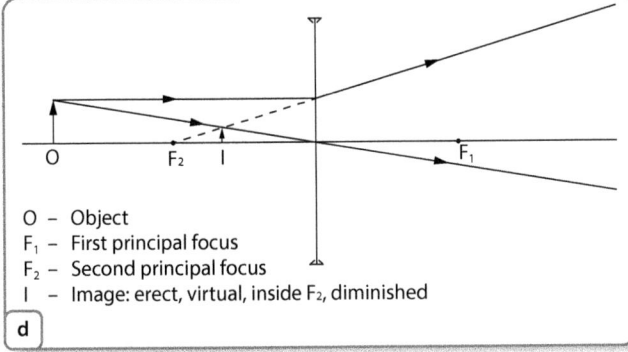

O – Object
F_1 – First principal focus
F_2 – Second principal focus
I – Image: erect, virtual, inside F_2, diminished

d

65. B 5 dioptres

Amplitude of accommodation is given by the formula:

$$A = P - R$$

where A is the amplitude of accommodation, P is the near point in dioptres and R is the far point in dioptres.

The dioptric power can be calculated as the reciprocal of the distance in metres. In this case:

$$P = \frac{1}{0.2} = 5 \text{ dioptres}$$

The far point in emmetropia is infinity, and for these purposes the reciprocal of infinity is taken as 0. Therefore, 5 − 0 = 5 dioptres of accommodation.

66. C Lux

Lux is photometric unit of illuminance, measured as lumen/m^2. Watt/m^2 are the equivalent radiometric units of irradiance.

67. B The cylinder in the cross cylinder has twice the power of the sphere

Jackson's cross cylinder is made up of a cylinder that is twice the power of the sphere, and of the opposite sign. Another way of describing it is a pair of cylindrical lenses with axes at 90° to each other. The handle is positioned between the two axes, so lies at 45° to each axis.

The cross cylinder allows testing of the axis and power of the cylindrical element during subjective refraction. Whilst checking the axis, the handle of the cross cylinder is held in line with the axis of the trial cylinder. Whilst checking the power, the positive or negative cylinder marking on the cross cylinder is held in line with the axis of the trial cylinder. When no cylindrical element has been found on retinoscopy, the cross cylinder can be used to confirm this.

68. B The angle of incidence equals the angle of emergence

In the Prentice position, a prism is placed such that the light ray is normal to one surface of the prism. All the deviation occurs on the far surface (**Figure 1.3**). Unlike in the position of minimum deviation, the angle of incidence does not equal the angle of emergence.

The Prentice position power is typically specified for glass prisms, whereas plastic ones are usually intended to be used in the position of minimum deviation. If a prism is held in the wrong position, its effective power changes.

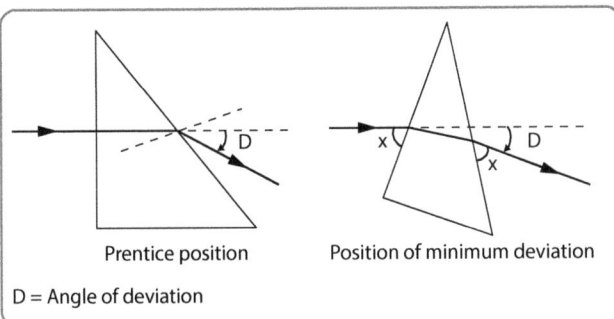

Figure 1.3 Angle of deviation at prisms: Prentice position vs. position of minimum deviation.

Prentice position   Position of minimum deviation

D = Angle of deviation

69. **D When a plane mirror is rotated by 45°, light reflected on the centre of rotation is deviated by 90°**

    The laws of reflection are as follows:

    - The angle of incidence equals the angle of reflection. Both angles are usually measured with respect to the normal to the reflecting surface
    - The incident and reflected rays, as well as the normal to the reflecting surface, are all in the same plane

    These are true regardless of the nature of the surface.

    Some reflection of light occurs at all interfaces, even if most of the light is transmitted, such as with a glass door.

    If light is reflected by a plane mirror that is rotated, the reflected ray is deviated by an angle twice as large as the angle of rotation. This is because both the angle of incidence and angle of reflection are increased by the angle of rotation.

70. **D Virtual, erect, laterally inverted**

    Reflection of an object at a plane (flat) mirror produces an image that is virtual, erect and laterally inverted (**Figure 1.4**). The object is in front of the mirror, and the image lies the same distance behind it, on a line perpendicular to the mirror. The image is neither enlarged nor diminished.

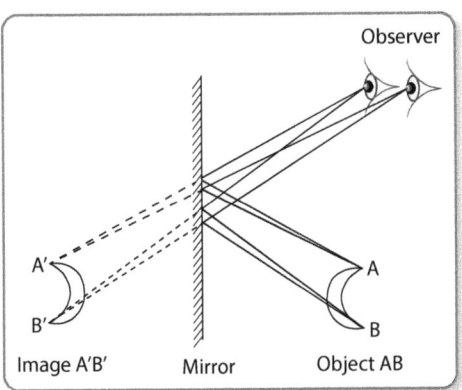

Figure 1.4 Reflection at a plane mirror.

71. **D** When light passes from air to Crown glass, the angles of incidence (*i*) and refraction (*r*) are related as follows:

$$1.52 = \frac{\cos i}{\cos r}$$

The correct relationship is:

$$1.52 = \frac{\sin i}{\sin r}$$

When passing into an optically denser medium, light is deviated towards the normal (the normal to the surface at the point of incidence). Conversely, when light enters an optically less dense medium, it is deviated away from the normal.

Snell's law describes the relationship between the optical densities of the two media and the angles of incidence (*i*) and refraction (*r*):

$$\frac{n_2}{n_1} = \frac{\sin i}{\sin r}$$

where n_1 is the refractive index of the first medium, and n_2 that of the second medium; and where the incident ray, refracted ray and the normal are all in the same plane.

When light passes from air (refractive index of 1) into another medium, the equation becomes:

$$\frac{n_2}{1} = \frac{\sin i}{\sin r}$$

The example in option (d) in the question, air to Crown glass (refractive index of 1.52), is therefore false, and should be as follows:

$$1.52 = \frac{\sin i}{\sin r}$$

72. **C −2.75 DS**

The spherical equivalent is the closest spherical lens power to a given toric lens. It is calculated by adding half the cylindrical power to that of the sphere.

In the example given, the spherical lens power is −3.50 with a +1.50 cylinder at axis 70°. The spherical equivalent of this is therefore:

$$-3.50 + ½ (+1.50) = -2.75$$

Option B is the correct transposition of this lens from positive to negative cylinder format, rather than the spherical equivalent.

73. **B 22.5 dioptre**

As a lens placed in the sulcus has effectively been moved further from the retina its effective power will increase, and so the power of the intraocular lens (IOL) must be reduced to compensate. Studies have shown that an adjustment of −1 dioptres is appropriate in eyes with a normal axial length. If the IOL power predicted for the capsular bag is greater than 28 dioptres then an adjustment of −1.5 would be appropriate. Similarly, if the IOL power predicted for the capsular bag is less than 17.5 dioptres then an adjustment of −0.5 would be appropriate. For very low IOL powers (below 9.5 dioptres) the IOL power should not be changed.

74. **C The glass of the Maddox rod is clear to eliminate chromatic aberration**

The glass of the Maddox rod is tinted (usually red) in order to give a coloured line to compare to the white dot seen with the other eye.

A white spot target is viewed with a Maddox rod over one eye. This should be at least 6 metres distant.

A line is seen through the Maddox rod at 90° to the axis of the rod. This is because the light parallel to the axis of the Maddox rod is unaffected by it, and therefore is focused on the retina normally, forming a row of foci at 90° to the axis (the row of foci formed are perceived as a line). Conversely the light at 90° to the axis is focused by the powerful convex cylindrical lenses of the rod and form a series of lines immediately in front of the eye that run parallel to the axis of the Maddox rod. The light from these lines is dispersing at a sharp angle when it reaches the cornea and it is thus out of focus at the retina.

75. **A Cardiff cards**

The Cardiff cards test is a preferential looking test of visual acuity aimed at toddlers aged 1–3 years, although it can also be used in older children or adults with intellectual impairment.

Frisby testing involves identifying the 'different' picture from a group of patterns on varying thicknesses of plate (one will have a hidden circle printed on the back surface only visible with stereopsis). It does not require special glasses, and can be used in young children.

The Titmus test (sometimes called the Wirt fly test as one of the key images is a housefly) involves looking at vectographs through polarised glasses. The composite image is seen if sufficient stereoacuity is present.

The Worth 4-dot test involves viewing four dots arranged in a diamond: two green, one red, and one white. Red/green goggles are worn. The number and position of the lights seen allow assessment of stereopsis and binocular function.

76. **A A patient's refractive error has a greater effect on indirect ophthalmoscopy**

A patient's refractive error has a greater effect on direct ophthalmoscopy. Direct ophthalmoscopy gives greater magnification (×15 in the emmetropic eye) than indirect ophthalmoscopy. Indirect ophthalmoscopy gives an image that is inverted vertically and horizontally, whereas direct ophthalmoscopy gives an erect image with no lateral inversion. The field of view is substantially greater with an indirect ophthalmoscope than with a direct ophthalmoscope. With the indirect ophthalmoscope, both the field of view and magnification vary according to the power of lens used.

77. **C One focal line is on the retina whilst the other is behind it**

   In simple astigmatism, one focal line falls on the retina whilst the other is either in front of or behind it. In simple hypermetropic astigmatism, the other focal line is behind the retina, as the eye does not have sufficient focusing power in that meridian.

   Compound astigmatism entails both focal lines falling either in front of or behind the retina. In mixed astigmatism, one focal line falls either side of the retina.

78. **C** $$\frac{+6.00 \text{ DS}}{-4.00 \text{ DC axis } 90°/-5.00 \text{ DC axis } 180°}$$

   Toric transposition allows a base curve for the prescription to be specified. The steps are as follows:

   1. Ensure the cylinder in your prescription is the same sign as the base curve. If not, transpose it
      i. In the question, both the cylinder (−1.00 DC) and the base curve (−4 D) are negative
   2. Work out the numerator in the final toric formula (the sphere): from the sphere in your prescription, subtract the base curve
      i. $+2.00 - (-4) = +6.00$
   3. Work out the denominator (the base curve, then the cylinder). The axis of the base curve is at 90° to the cylinder in your prescription. The final cylinder is obtained by adding the base curve power to the cylinder
      i. The base curve is −4.00 D axis 90°
      ii. The cylinder is $-4 + (-1) = -5.00$ DC axis 180°

      iii. Put it all together: $$\frac{+6.00 \text{ DS}}{-4.00 \text{ DC axis } 90°/-5.00 \text{ DC axis } 180°}$$

79. **D 30 D**

   In indirect ophthalmoscopy the field of view increases with increasing power of examination lens, while the magnification decreases. The 15D lens is used for high magnification viewing of the posterior pole, while the 28D lens is often used in paediatrics where a wide field of view in a snap-shot is useful (it is also useful in patients with smaller pupils). 20D lenses are useful in general examination. 30D lenses are mostly used for patients with small pupils.

80. **A Virtual, erect, magnified, at infinity**

The Galilean telescope produces a virtual, erect, magnified image at infinity. The lenses within the telescope (a convex objective lens and a concave eyepiece lens) are separated by the difference between their focal lengths. The image formed can be shown in the ray diagram **Figure 1.5**.

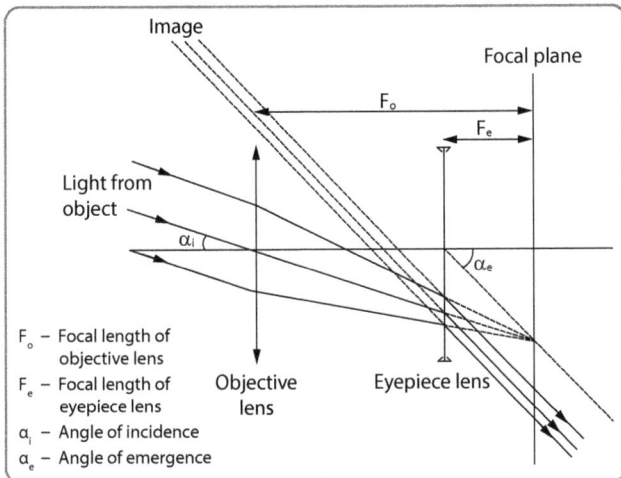

Figure 1.5 Galilean telescope.

81. **C The energy of a photon is directly proportional to its wavelength**

The energy of a photon is inversely proportional to its wavelength. The energy of a photon is defined by the equation:

$$E = h\nu$$

where E is the energy of a photon in joules, h is Planck's constant and ν is the frequency of the photon in hertz.

Therefore, the energy of a photon is directly proportional to its frequency. Frequency is related to wavelength by the equation:

$$\nu = \frac{c}{\lambda}$$

where c is the speed of light in a vacuum and λ is the wavelength in metres, hence the energy of a photon is inversely proportional to its wavelength.

Another consequence of the above equation relating energy to frequency (and therefore wavelength) is that as some of the energy from the excitation light in fluorescence reactions is converted to thermal or chemical energy the light emitted will have a lower energy, and therefore a lower frequency and longer wavelength. This can be seen with fluorescein, which reacts to a cobalt blue excitation light (485–500 nm) and emits a yellow-green light (525–530 nm).

Shorter wavelengths undergo increased scatter when compared with longer wavelengths. When caused by particles in a colloid or fine suspension this is known as the Tyndall effect, and causes the substance to appear blue (a common example is blue irides).

The wavelength of light decreases when travelling into a material with a higher refractive index. As the absolute refractive index of a material is defined as the ratio of the speed of light in a vacuum to the speed of light in the material we can see that the speed of light decreases on entering any material with a higher refractive index. The frequency of a wave does not change on moving from one material to another, and therefore as the speed of light decreases the wavelength of light decreases by the same factor.

82. A Destructive interference is used in anti-reflection coatings

Anti-reflection coatings are classically designed so that their thickness is roughly a quarter of the wavelength of incident light. Therefore, the reflected light from the film and the reflected light from the coated surface will be half a wavelength out of phase with each other, and hence produce destructive interference. Modern low-reflective coatings are often made up of several thin layers, but they still use the principle of destructive interference for their effect.

Laser light generates interference more readily than conventional light as it is closer to true monochromatic light. This property is used in laser interferometry.

The corneal stroma uses destructive interference in maintaining clarity. The collagen bundles are regularly spaced so that scattered light is eliminated by destructive interference.

Two waves of equal amplitude need to be out of phase by half a cycle to cancel each other out by destructive interference.

83. D Time spent outdoors as a child is a protective factor against myopia

The prevalence of myopia worldwide varies considerably with ethnicity and geographical distribution, being particularly high in Southeast and East Asians compared to other ethnicities.

Children are born relatively hypermetropic, which is overcome by their large amplitude of accommodation, and emmetropisation occurs as the eye grows. The prevalence of myopia is therefore higher in older children and adults than in young children.

Many factors affect emmetropisation. Risk factors for myopia include genetic and environmental factors. A family history of myopia and high level of educational attainment are risk factors for myopia, whilst time spent outdoors in childhood is a protective factor. Low dose atropine has been used in children to slow the rate of progression of myopia.

Pathology

84. D Renal cell carcinoma

Acoustic neuromas (also known as vestibular schwannomas) are principally a feature of neurofibromatosis type 2 (NF2), and nearly all patients with NF2 will develop them before the age of 30 (typically bilaterally). However, they can also occur unilaterally in neurofibromatosis type 1 (NF1).

NF2 is associated with meningioma.

The *NF1* gene is on chromosome 17; the *NF2* gene is on chromosome 22. Both are autosomal dominant. The name neurofibromatosis is a misnomer in the case of NF2, as the principal tumour types are neuromas (schwannomas) and meningiomas.

Phaeochromocytomas occur in NF1, as well as in Von Hippel–Lindau syndrome (VHL). Renal cell carcinomas occur in VHL, but are not associated with neurofibromatosis (although, as tumour suppressor genes, mutations in *NF1* and *NF2* are sometimes seen in renal cell carcinoma cells).

85. D Sympathetic ophthalmia

Dalen–Fuchs nodules are groups of epithelioid cells (activated macrophages) and lymphocytes between Bruch's membrane and the retinal pigment epithelium. They are a result of granulomatous inflammation at this site and can be seen in sympathetic ophthalmia, and also in other rare conditions including Vogt–Koyanagi–Harada (VKH) syndrome.

86. A 12%

Uveal tract melanomas may occur in the iris, ciliary body or choroid. Approximately 8% will occur in the iris, 12% in the ciliary body and 80% in the choroid. This is roughly equivalent to the relative tissue volumes of these structures.

87. D There is characteristic muscle wasting, often involving facial and extraocular muscles

Although myasthenia frequently causes weakness and fatigability in facial, bulbar and extraocular muscles, it does not characteristically cause muscle wasting. The muscle weakness can be temporarily improved with an ice pack applied for 5 minutes. This has been proposed to be due to the inhibition of acetylcholinesterase at low temperatures. A Tensilon test may also be used. Cogan's lid twitch is seen when the patient returns to the primary position from downgaze. The upper lid initially overshoots, then 'twitches' downwards.

88. B Hyperplasia

Hyperplasia refers to an increase in the number of cells in a tissue. Hypertrophy refers to an increase in the size of individual cells. Both of these processes can cause a tissue to enlarge. Metaplasia refers to the change of differentiated cells to another cell type (this may be a less differentiated cell type). Dysplasia of cells refers to the proliferation of abnormal (often immature) cells in a tissue.

89. **A Amyloid appears as a homogenous blue material on haematoxylin and eosin (H&E) staining**

    Amyloid is an insoluble fibrous protein and therefore takes up the pink eosin stain in an H&E stain, rather than the blue haematoxylin which binds to acidic structures such as nucleic acids. In lattice dystrophy, amyloid deposits are seen in the corneal stroma. Systemic amyloidosis is significantly more common than localised amyloidosis. Amyloid exhibits 'apple' green birefringence when exposed to polarised light after staining with Congo red.

90. **D Outer plexiform layer**

    Hard exudates are caused by localised hypoperfusion, leading to damage to the endothelium of deep capillaries and breakdown of the inner blood–retinal barrier. This causes leakage of plasma into the outer plexiform layer of the retina, leading to what appear clinically as discrete, pale yellow deposits. Histologically, these stain pink on H&E, and contain foamy macrophages.

91. **D Unilateral**

    Corneal arcus occurs most commonly as part of the normal ageing process, but is also seen in hyperlipidaemia. It is a fatty degeneration of the peripheral cornea that causes a circumferential opacity near the limbal margin. Lipid deposition occurs in the stroma. It is a bilateral condition: unilateral arcus is very rare, and causes include ocular ischaemia and hypotony.

92. **A Accumulation of subretinal fluid occurs in all types of retinal detachment**

    Retinal detachment is a separation of the neurosensory retina from the retinal pigment epithelium. There are three main types of retinal detachment (**Table 1.7**), all of which involve the accumulation of subretinal fluid. Rhegmatogenous is the most common.

Table 1.7 Types of retinal detachment		
Type	Pathophysiology	Common causes
Rhegmatogenous	Liquefaction of vitreous, vitreoretinal traction, retinal tear or break	• Posterior vitreous detachment causing retinal tear or hole • Dehiscence of the anterior retina at the ora serrata causing retinal dialysis (usually due to trauma)
Exudative/Serous	Compromised outer blood–retinal barrier	• Vascular, e.g. wet age-related macular degeneration • Inflammatory, e.g. posterior scleritis • Neoplastic, e.g. choroidal melanoma
Tractional	Contracting proliferative retinal membranes, abnormal vitreoretinal adhesions	• Proliferative diabetic retinopathy • Proliferative vitreoretinopathy • Retinopathy of prematurity

93. C Raised intraocular pressure is common, due to inflammation

Proliferative vitreoretinopathy is a common cause of failure following retinal detachment surgery and is more common with large breaks, multiple operations and duration of retinal detachment. It may also occur in untreated retinal detachment. Following the break in the retina, retinal pigment epithelial cells migrate into the subretinal space and vitreous. The blood–retinal barrier is broken and inflammatory cells are recruited. Fibrosis and collagen production occur, contributing to the formation of retinal membranes. Contraction of these can lead to retinal detachment and, if untreated, ocular hypotony (not raised intraocular pressure) and ultimately phthisis bulbi.

94. B Regeneration of the epithelium and Bowman's layer

Bowman's layer does not regenerate. The phases of healing of a full-thickness corneal laceration are listed in **Table 1.8**.

Table 1.8 Phases of healing of a full-thickness corneal laceration	
Time	Phase of healing
Minutes	Retraction of Descemet's membrane and stromal collagen Fibrin plug formation Stromal oedema Invasion of leucocytes from aqueous and limbal vessels
Hours	Transformation of leucocytes and stromal keratocytes into fibroblasts Collagen formation Start of epithelial regeneration
Days	Endothelial sliding, filling in gaps in endothelium and Descemet's membrane
Weeks	Replacement of stroma and Bowman's layer with scar tissue

Pharmacology

95. A Brief blockade of synaptic transmission

Botulinum toxin A is a potent neurotoxin which inhibits the release of acetylcholine at the neuromuscular junction. It achieves this by cleaving SNARE proteins, which are required for fusion of the neurosecretory vesicles with the plasma membrane, thus blocking the exocytosis of acetylcholine. It causes long-lasting blockade of synaptic transmission. Botulinum toxin poisoning is characterised by progressive parasympathetic and motor paralysis. Botulinum toxin A is used therapeutically in ophthalmology by local injection into muscles in the treatment of blepharospasm, hemifacial spasm and strabismus, and to induce ptosis.

96. D Lipid-soluble drugs can pass the blood–retinal barrier

Drugs absorbed from the gastrointestinal tract pass through the portal circulation before reaching the systemic circulation and may be metabolised by the liver in a process known as first-pass metabolism. Although eye drops often have few systemic side effects, this is not always the case as any drug absorbed systemically via the nasopharyngeal mucosa avoids first pass metabolism.

The metabolism of drugs can be described in terms of first- or zero-order kinetics. First-order kinetics are linear where the rate is proportional to the concentration of drug. In zero-order kinetics, the metabolism of the drug is independent of the concentration (non-linear).

Drug distribution depends on several factors including protein binding and lipid solubility. Highly protein-bound drugs tend to remain in the plasma compartment. In general, lipid solubility increases drug absorption and distribution, for example by allowing diffusion across cell membranes and the blood–retinal barrier.

97. A Bone marrow suppression

Ciclosporin, along with tacrolimus, is a calcineurin inhibitor whose immunosuppressant effects are via action on T lymphocytes. It inhibits the transcription of IL-2 and other cytokines. Side effects include nephrotoxicity, tremor, hirsutism, and gingival hypertrophy.

98. B Hydroxyamphetamine 1%

The working diagnosis in this patient is Horner's syndrome secondary to a Pancoast tumour in the pulmonary apex. This is a preganglionic lesion affecting the second-order neuron.

Failure to dilate to cocaine is diagnostic of Horner's syndrome regardless of the level of the lesion. Cocaine inhibits the reuptake of noradrenaline at sympathetic synapses, so has no effect if no noradrenaline is secreted. In this patient, the right pupil should fail to dilate to cocaine.

Failure to dilate to hydroxyamphetamine indicates a postganglionic lesion, i.e. affecting the third-order neuron. This is because it causes release of noradrenaline from postganglionic nerve terminals which can only occur with an intact third order neuron. In this patient, both pupils should dilate.

These agents are learnt for exams but are not usually available in a modern eye clinic. Apraclonidine and dilute phenylephrine (1%) have been used as alternatives (**Table 1.9**), although the positive reaction in Horner's is a dilatation,

Table 1.9 Pharmacological agents used in the diagnosis of Horner's syndrome			
Positive result	Agent	Level of lesion	Mechanism
Fails to dilate	Cocaine 4%	All Horner's	Inhibits NA reuptake at sympathetic synapses, so no effect if no NA secreted
	Hydroxyamphetamine 1%	3rd order lesion	Stimulates release of NA from post-ganglionic nerve terminals
Dilates, i.e. reversal of anisocoria	Apraclonidine 0.5% or 1%	All Horner's	α_2 agonist with weak α_1 activity Denervation hypersensitivity
	Phenylephrine 1%	3rd order lesion	α_1 agonist Denervation hypersensitivity
(NA: noradrenaline)			

rather than a failure to dilate. Note that denervation hypersensitivity to apraclonidine is due to upregulation of iris α_1 receptors and may take several days to develop. Thus, a negative apraclonidine test in the acute setting does not exclude Horner's syndrome.

Pilocarpine constricts rather than dilates the pupil so is not helpful.

99. A α_2 agonist

Brimonidine is an α_2 adrenoreceptor agonist which lowers aqueous production as well as increasing uveoscleral outflow.

The four possible answers listed are the principal classes of topical medication used in the treatment of open angle glaucoma and ocular hypertension. The pros and cons of each drop must be weighed up for an individual patient when making treatment decisions. When compared to the other classes, α_2 agonists such as brimonidine carry more risk of allergy (~10%). However, they are considered safer than the other classes in pregnancy, and they are not contraindicated in asthma (unlike beta-blockers).

100. A Hyperkalaemia

Acetazolamide is a carbonic anhydrase inhibitor used as a systemic intraocular pressure-lowering agent.

Patients commonly experience paraesthesia of the extremities. Additionally, serious side effects of acetazolamide include hypokalaemia and potassium depletion, metabolic acidosis, renal stones, depression; and more rarely, blood disorders and Stevens–Johnson syndrome.

Due to this side effect profile, long term use of acetazolamide is not generally recommended. However, it is highly valuable in gaining control of intraocular pressure in certain situations, for example in the management of acute angle closure.

101. D Thromboxane A_2 causes vasoconstriction

Eicosanoids are an important group of signalling molecules and inflammatory mediators that include prostaglandins and thromboxanes (together termed prostanoids), and leukotrienes. They can be generated as required in response to stimuli. The inflammatory response always involves prostanoid generation.

The precise stimuli vary depending on cell type and include cell damage, thrombin (platelets), complement-derived C5a (neutrophils) and bradykinin (fibroblasts). They are derived from polyunsaturated fatty acids, principally arachidonic acid, which is liberated from cell membrane phospholipids in a rate-limiting step catalysed primarily by phospholipase A_2. The enzymes cyclooxygenase (COX-1 and COX-2 isoforms) and lipoxygenase then catalyse the production of different eicosanoids from free arachidonic acid.

Nonsteroidal anti-inflammatory drugs (NSAIDs) reduce inflammation by inhibiting cyclooxygenase, and therefore the biosynthesis of prostaglandins, but subsequently have no effect on their actions on target tissue. Prostaglandins exert their effects by acting on G-protein-coupled receptors.

Thromboxane A_2 is an eicosanoid which causes vasoconstriction and platelet aggregation.

102. C Midazolam

Benzodiazepines are used for sedation, premedication and induction of anaesthesia, and as anxiolytics, anticonvulsants and muscle relaxants. They act on the $GABA_A$ receptor in the central nervous system.

The half-lives of different benzodiazepines, outlined in **Table 1.10**, are a key factor in determining their use. Whilst the exact half-lives need not be memorised (and vary between published sources) it is important to know, for example, that midazolam is short acting, making it suitable for sedation for short procedures and induction.

Table 1.10 Half-lives of different benzodiazepines	
Benzodiazepine	**Half-life (hours)**
Midazolam	1–3
Temazepam	6–8
Lorazepam	12
Diazepam	12–24

Physiology

103. C Increased vascular permeability

Histamine exerts its physiological effects by acting on histamine receptors, of which there are four types: H_1, H_2, H_3, and H_4. They are all G-protein-coupled receptors. Histamine is an inflammatory mediator and its effects in type I hypersensitivity reactions are via the H_1 receptor. Its gastric effects are mainly H_2-mediated, along with its effects on Th1 lymphocyte cytokine production. H_3 receptors are expressed mainly in the central nervous system and affect the release of various neurotransmitters. H_4 receptors are found in large numbers on immune cells, including mast cells, eosinophils and dendritic cells, and when activated they amplify the histamine-mediated inflammatory response through their role in chemotaxis and the release of inflammatory mediators.

Histamine is released during mast cell degranulation, and can modulate degranulation, but this is via action on H_4 receptors. Some important actions of histamine via the H_1 and H_2 histamine receptors are shown in **Table 1.11**.

Table 1.11 Histamine receptors		
Receptor	Intracellular effects	Physiological effects
H_1 receptor	Activation of phospholipase C Increased intracellular calcium concentration	• Increased vascular permeability • Vasodilatation • Central nervous system depression
H_2 receptor	Activation of adenylate cyclase and increase in cAMP	• Increased gastric acid production • Increased cardiac stroke volume

104. B Chromaticity is an objective measure of colour quality

Chromaticity is an objective measurement of colour quality, defined by its hue and saturation.

Retinal sensitivity to different colours changes with the level of illumination. As illumination decreases the peak sensitivity of the retina shifts towards blue, causing red colours to appear darker and the visual environment to appear more blue. This is called the Purkinje effect, and occurs in mesopic conditions due to the increasing influence of rod photoreceptors (peak sensitivity of 498 nm).

The maximal spectral sensitivity of green cones is 535–550 nm (see table on page 151).

Perception of hue is also dependent on the level of illuminance. With increasing illumination, longer wavelengths appear more yellow, and shorter wavelengths appear more blue. This is known as the Bezold–Brücke effect.

105. C Increased cone sensitivity accounts for the early component of the dark adaptation curve

Dark adaptation is the process by which the retina increases in sensitivity to light in response to decreasing background illumination.

The dark adaptation curve plots the light intensity required to perceive a spot of light versus time. It is bipartite, with an initial rapid (5–10 minutes) increase in cone sensitivity and then a slower period (15–30 minutes) where rods reach their maximum sensitivity. Thus dark adaptation is complete in 30 minutes in normal subjects.

Fully dark-adapted rods allow perception of a spot of light at least 100 times dimmer than cones can perceive.

Light adaptation occurs more rapidly than dark adaptation.

106. B Insulin promotes the movement of potassium from the intracellular to the extracellular compartment

Insulin promotes uptake of potassium by cells, therefore movement from the extracellular to the intracellular compartment.

Potassium is the chief intracellular cation, with an intracellular fluid concentration of approximately 135–150 mmol/L (versus 3.5–5 mmol/L in extracellular fluid, aqueous and plasma). This gradient is largely maintained by the Na$^+$/K$^+$-ATPase pump. Over 90% of total body potassium is intracellular.

Daily potassium requirements are approximately 1 mmol/kg/day. Renal handling of potassium is crucial in maintaining potassium homeostasis. Potassium is reabsorbed at the proximal convoluted tubule and then secreted back into the urine by the distal convoluted tubule (promoted by aldosterone). Renal potassium excretion is also influenced by antidiuretic hormone (ADH), tubular flow rate and acid–base balance.

107. B Atrial contraction is responsible for 80% of ventricular filling

The cardiac cycle is divided into five phases (**Table 1.12**).

Table 1.12 Phases of the cardiac cycle		
1	Atrial systole	
2	Isometric ventricular contraction	Ventricular systole
3	Ventricular contraction	
4	Isometric ventricular relaxation	Diastole
5	Ventricular filling	

Although contraction of the two sides of the heart occurs during the same phases of the cardiac cycle, it is slightly asynchronous:

- Right atrial contraction begins before left
- Left ventricular contraction begins before right

Rapid passive filling of the ventricles occurs in early diastole. Atrial contraction is responsible for only 30% of ventricular filling.

On an electrocardiography (ECG) trace of the cardiac cycle, the P wave corresponds to atrial depolarisation.

108. B Somatostatin promotes the release of growth hormone from the anterior pituitary

The hypothalamus secretes releasing or release-inhibiting hormones which act on the pituitary gland. These are sometimes referred to as 'factors', e.g. corticotrophin-releasing factor (CRF), thyrotrophin-releasing factor (TRF) and growth hormone-release-inhibiting factor (better known as somatostatin).

The actions of growth hormone, secreted by the anterior pituitary, include increased skeletal growth, protein synthesis, gluconeogenesis and lipolysis. The effects of over-secretion depend on whether it occurs before puberty (gigantism) or after puberty (acromegaly).

The secretion of hormones from the anterior pituitary, including growth hormone and adrenocorticotropic hormone (ACTH), is pulsatile.

Answers: SBAs

109. B Oncotic pressure

Oncotic pressure is generated by plasma proteins and works against aqueous humour production. Recall that the aqueous is virtually free of protein in the healthy state. Production of aqueous is maintained by active secretion in the double-layered ciliary epithelium, passive diffusion of ions down their concentration and charge gradients, and ultrafiltration of water and solutes secondary to the capillary hydrostatic pressure. Of these processes active secretion is thought to account for 80–90% of aqueous humour production.

110. D 4

The primary visual cortex (V1), like all cerebral cortical areas, is divided into six basic layers. The neurons of the optic radiations travel from the lateral geniculate nucleus to layer 4 of the primary visual cortex and synapse there. Layer 4 of the primary visual cortex is expanded into distinct sub-layers with a central white line known as the stria of Gennari. This represents the myelinated fibres of the optic radiations. It is because of this appearance of distinct sub-layers that the primary visual cortex is sometimes referred to as the striate cortex.

111. B Cells in layer 5 project principally to the secondary visual cortex

Cells in layer 5 project to the superior colliculus. Input to the secondary visual cortex is by layers 2 and 3. Layer 6 provides feed-forward innervation to the lateral geniculate nucleus. The superior lip of the calcarine sulcus receives input from the superior retina (and therefore the inferior visual field), and vice versa for the inferior lip of the sulcus. There are alternating ocular dominance columns in layer 4 C, each responsive to inputs from a single eye. Thus neurons corresponding to each eye are segregated as far as the primary visual cortex.

112. B Circadian rhythm

The suprachiasmatic nucleus receives input from the retina via the retinohypothalamic tract and generates the circadian rhythm cycle via the action of pacemaker cells. These influence the production of melatonin in the pineal gland, which in turn allows physiological adjustment to the light–dark cycle. As the light–dark cycle changes during the course of the year the suprachiasmatic nucleus permits the organisation of physiological functions on both a diurnal and a seasonal basis.

A summary of subcortical structures related to vision is given in Table 3.9 (page 229).

113. D Keratan sulphate

All of these glycosaminoglycans are found in the cornea, but keratan sulphate is thought to be crucial for maintaining corneal clarity. It binds to collagen arrays and is thought to maintain interfibrillar distance.

114. D The magnitude of an action potential determines the quantity of neurotransmitter released

Action potentials are an 'all-or-nothing' response, in that when they are initiated they will always obtain the same magnitude. Information is instead transmitted by the number of action potentials and their frequency.

The cell membranes of neurons usually have a negatively charged resting membrane potential, which can be depolarised by various stimuli (for example the opening of ligand-gated ion channels on their dendrites). The cell membranes of neurons contain voltage-gated sodium channels which will allow an influx of Na^+ ions when a threshold voltage is reached. This further depolarises the cell, generating a feedback loop and triggering an action potential. Once the cell is depolarised the voltage-gated sodium channels close and voltage-gated potassium channels open. This causes an outward flow of K^+ ions, repolarising the cell membrane. The density of voltage-gated sodium channels is highest at the initial segment of the axon (the axon hillock for motor neurons and interneurons, and the first node of Ranvier for myelinated sensory neurons), and so this is where action potentials are generally triggered.

115. C Vergence movements

Disconjugate movements are when both eyes move in opposite directions, and are seen in vergence movements where the eyes either converge or diverge. Other eye movements are conjugate, i.e. both eyes move in the same direction. Key eye movements are listed below in **Table 1.13**.

Table 1.13 Key eye movements	
Eye movement	**Key features**
Saccade	Rapid ballistic movement to change point of fixation Voluntary or reflexive May be small (e.g. when reading) or large (e.g. looking up from your desk) Maximum velocity ~900°/second
Smooth pursuit	Slow tracking movement to keep a target on the fovea Voluntary movement (although requires a moving stimulus) Maximum velocity ~100°/second
Vergence	Disconjugate movement (convergence or divergence) Generally used to change between near and distance focus points Uses retinal disparity to calculate movement required Part of the accommodation response Slower than smooth pursuit movement
Vestibulo-ocular	Stabilise the eye relative to the external world Rapid movements to compensate for changes in head position Reflex movement Independent of visual input

116. C Right inferior oblique and left superior oblique

Yoked muscles are pairs of extraocular muscles designed to bring about a co-ordinated direction of gaze. Each medial rectus is paired with the opposite lateral rectus, each superior oblique is paired with the opposite inferior rectus and each inferior oblique is paired with the opposite superior rectus.

117. A Ciliary muscle relaxation

The ciliary muscle contracts during accommodation, allowing an increase in lens curvature and therefore refractive power. The eyes converge to focus on the near target and the pupil constricts to restrict the passage of light to the central lens.

118. A Depolarisation of hair cells in the cochlea occurs due to the influx of sodium

Unlike most other excitable tissues, depolarisation in the hair cell occurs due to an influx of potassium (not sodium) from the endolymph.

Sound waves cause vibrations of the tympanic membrane, which are transmitted and magnified across the middle ear by the ossicles to the inner ear. Vibrations in the endolymph cause vibrations in the basilar membrane of the cochlea which is where the organ of Corti is located. The organ of Corti transduces the vibrations into action potentials in the auditory nerve.

Sound is audible to humans between approximately 20 and 20,000 Hz, with the greatest sensitivity being in the 1,000–4,000 Hz range. Different pitches stimulate hair cells at different locations in the organ of Corti. Higher frequencies are detected by hair cells near the base of the cochlea, and low tones near the apex.

Statistics and evidence-based medicine

119. C 70%

Sensitivity is a statistical value which measures the ability of a test to correctly assign a positive outcome to a patient. It is defined as the probability of the test being positive when the disease is present. It can be calculated by the formula below:

$$\text{Sensitivity} = \frac{x}{x+y}$$

where x is the number of true positives (tested positive and found to be positive) and y is the number of false negatives (tested negative and found to be positive).

In this case:

$$\text{Sensitivity} = \frac{35}{35+15} = 70\%$$

120. A Failing to reject the null hypothesis when it is false

A type II error is when a study fails to reject the null hypothesis even though it is false, i.e. failing to detect a real difference. Conversely a type I error is where a null hypothesis is rejected when it is true, i.e. finding a difference when there is none.

Answers: CRQs

Anatomy

1. Answer

(a) The diagram shows a coronal section through the cavernous sinus, midway along the body of the sphenoid bone. Inferior to the cavernous sinus are the sphenoid air spaces (unlabelled), and above it the optic chiasm (not pictured). The labelled structures are:

A. Maxillary division of trigeminal nerve (V2)

B. Ophthalmic division of trigeminal nerve (V1)

C. Abducens nerve (VI)

D. Internal carotid artery

E. Trochlear nerve (IV)

F. Oculomotor nerve (III)

G. Pituitary gland (hypophysis cerebri)

(b) Two conditions which typically affect the cavernous sinus are:

Carotid–cavernous fistula (arteriovenous fistula also acceptable)
Cavernous sinus thrombosis (venous thrombosis also acceptable)

Feedback
A carotid–cavernous fistula is an abnormal arteriovenous communication between the internal carotid artery and the cavernous sinus, resulting in arterialisation of the venous flow with raised venous pressure and venous stasis. Carotid–cavernous fistulae may be traumatic, spontaneous (usually elderly patients) or congenital. They may be direct, high-flow shunts, presenting with a red eye with pulsatile proptosis; or indirect, low-flow shunts where the arteriovenous communication is at the level of smaller branches of the carotid arteries, with more subtle clinical features.

The superior and inferior ophthalmic veins and the facial vein all communicate with the cavernous sinus. Thus infection of the facial skin, orbit or paranasal sinuses may lead to the spread of septic emboli and resulting cavernous sinus thrombosis. Noninfectious cavernous sinus thrombosis also occurs (often with a more subtle presentation), with risk factors including prothrombotic states such as malignancy and oral contraceptive use. The clinical features of cavernous sinus thrombosis depend on the structures affected and are caused by venous congestion, cranial nerve involvement or any underlying infection.

(c) The abducens nerve (VI)

Feedback
The abducens nerve (VI) is the most vulnerable due to its intraluminal course through the cavernous sinus. The other cranial nerves pass along the wall of the sinus which offers a degree of protection; III, IV, and V nerve involvement is therefore less common.

Biochemistry and cell biology

2. Answer

(a) Synaptic vesicles

Feedback
Neurotransmitter molecules at the synaptic terminal are stored in synaptic vesicles (also known as presynaptic vesicles) prior to release.

(b) Noradrenaline (norepinephrine) *(1 mark for either name)*

Feedback
Postganglionic sympathetic fibres release noradrenaline (also called norepinephrine) as their principal neurotransmitter, except the neurons innervating the adrenal medulla and the post-ganglionic sympathetic neurons of sweat glands.

(c) Tyrosine

Feedback
Tyrosine (or 4-hydroxyphenylalanine) is converted to L-DOPA by the enzyme tyrosine hydroxylase. L-DOPA is then converted to dopamine by DOPA decarboxylase. Dopamine β-hydroxylase converts dopamine into noradrenaline.

(d) Dopamine and adrenaline (epinephrine) *(1 mark for each)*

Feedback
As described above, dopamine is the metabolic precursor to noradrenaline, and is an important neurotransmitter in several systems in the central nervous system. Adrenaline (also called epinephrine) is synthesised from noradrenaline by the action of phenylethanolamine N-methyltransferase (PNMT), and acts as a neurotransmitter as well as a circulating hormone.

(e) Exocytosis

Feedback
Neurotransmitters are released by exocytosis. The synaptic vesicles containing neurotransmitter molecules fuse with the cell membrane at the synaptic terminal, releasing neurotransmitter into the synaptic cleft.

(f) Metabotropic (G-protein-coupled) receptors and ionotropic (ligand-gated ion channel) receptors. Metabotropic (G-protein-coupled) receptors are responsible for transmission at this synapse. *(1 mark for each type of receptor, mark given if either nomenclature used, and a further mark for correctly identifying the type at this synapse)*

Feedback
The two classes of receptors found at synapses are metabotropic (G-protein-coupled) receptors, which exert their influence by activating an intracellular G protein which in turn modulates other intracellular signalling molecules; and ionotropic (ligand-gated ion channel) receptors, which incorporate an ion channel which will open or close depending on the binding of different ligands (e.g. a neurotransmitter). Non-G-protein-coupled metabotropic receptors can be found elsewhere as receptors for hormones, cytokines, and growth factors (e.g. receptor tyrosine kinases).

The principal post-synaptic receptors at this synapse are a_1 adrenoreceptors, which, like all adrenoreceptors, are G-protein-coupled.

(g) Acetylcholine

Feedback
Preganglionic sympathetic nerves, including those entering the superior cervical ganglion, release acetylcholine as their principal neurotransmitter. This acts on nicotinic acetylcholine receptors on the postganglionic sympathetic nerves.

Genetics

3. Answer

(a)

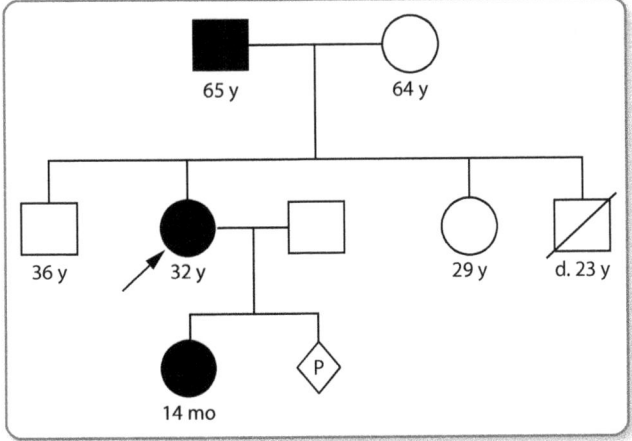

(5 marks for accurate pedigree, indicating proband, affected individuals, gender, deceased individual, pregnancy)

Feedback
The standardised rules and symbols for pedigree drawing include the following:

A square denotes a male individual; a circle denotes a female; and a diamond an individual of unknown sex.

It is good practice to write their age or year of birth underneath. Do not write the age in the symbol; this is used for multiple individuals, e.g. a circle with the number 5 in it indicates 5 unaffected females. Siblings should appear in age order with the eldest on the left.

The symbol is coloured in to denote affected individuals.

A marriage or partnership is indicated by a horizontal line between two symbols. A double horizontal line indicates a consanguineous marriage.

An arrow denotes the proband.

A pregnancy is indicated by a P within the symbol.

Deceased individuals are indicated by a diagonal line through their symbol.

(b) Autosomal dominant

Feedback
The features shown here that are characteristic of autosomal dominant inheritance are: affected individuals in each generation, both males and females affected, and multiple forms of transmission of the affected gene (male to female, female to female).

(c) 50%, the risk is the same for a boy or a girl

Feedback
In autosomal dominant conditions, there is a 50% risk of each child being affected, and the risk is not affected by the sex of the child. This assumes that the affected parent is a heterozygote for the gene in question, and the partner is unaffected. In this example, we know that this is the case as the proband's mother and husband are unaffected.

The risk is affected by the sex of the child in X-linked conditions. Most X-linked conditions are X-linked recessive. These conditions almost exclusively affect males (they can rarely affect females due to either the phenomenon of X-inactivation or the rare possibility of an affected father and a mother who is a carrier). As a father only passes on the Y chromosome to his son, the gene is passed on to males via the mother. Therefore, on a pedigree only female to male transmission is seen. All of an affected father's daughters will be carriers of the gene.

(d) Aniridia

Feedback
Aniridia is characterised by a spectrum of iris hypoplasia, ranging from

transillumination defects in the iris to near-complete absence of the iris. This is often accompanied by foveal hypoplasia (and/or optic nerve hypoplasia), which tends to cause pendular nystagmus and poor vision.

In aniridia, as well as in iridocorneal dysgenesis conditions such as Peters' anomaly and Axenfeld–Rieger syndrome, glaucoma occurs in over 50% of individuals. This is due to abnormalities in the trabecular meshwork. Other complications of aniridia include keratopathy secondary to limbal stem cell failure, and cataracts.

(e) *PAX6*

Feedback
Aniridia is caused by mutations or deletions affecting the *PAX6* gene on chromosome 11. It shows autosomal dominant inheritance, with high penetrance and variable expression. It is inherited in 2/3 of cases, with the remaining 1/3 being the result of *de novo* mutations. Aniridia can be an isolated condition, or, less commonly, can occur as part of a syndrome. For example, a deletion involving the short arm of chromosome 11 may affect the adjacent *WT1* tumour suppressor gene. This can lead to WAGR syndrome, consisting of Wilms' tumour (nephroblastoma), Aniridia, Genitourinary malformations, and mental Retardation (now more commonly referred to as intellectual disability, or general learning disability). Aniridia is also a feature of the rare Gillespie syndrome (aniridia, cerebellar ataxia, hypotonia, and intellectual disability), which can be autosomal recessive (See also feedback to Paper 2, SBA 39 on page 130).

Investigations and imaging

4. Answer

(a) Macular OCT (optical coherence tomography) scan

(b) A broadband, low coherence light source is directed at the desired target *(1 mark)*. A beam splitter is used to simultaneously direct the same light source at a reference mirror *(1 mark)*. The reflected light from both the desired target and the reference mirror are directed onto a detector, and the interference pattern is analysed using low coherence interferometry to construct an image of the desired target *(1 mark)*

(c) Any two of: it requires transparent media; it requires patient co-operation; it requires at least moderate dilatation; it is susceptible to motion artefact *(1 mark for each, up to 2 marks)*

(d) Cystoid macular oedema

Feedback
There is an abnormal accumulation of fluid in cystoid spaces within the inner retina. The most common site of fluid accumulation is the outer plexiform layer, most probably because this is the watershed area between the choroidal and retinal circulations.

(e) Any two of: postoperative inflammation, especially after cataract extraction (Irvine-Gass syndrome); uveitis; retinitis (e.g. CMV retinitis); diabetic maculopathy; retinal vein occlusion; vitreomacular traction (although not present in this scan); retinitis pigmentosa; topical adrenaline or prostaglandin E2 therapy; nicotinic acid therapy; niacin therapy; age-related macular degeneration *(1 mark for each, up to 2 marks)*

Feedback
Cystoid macular oedema is a shared pathological response to a number of inflammatory and retinal vascular processes. It can lead to blurred and/or distorted central vision, and remains a significant cause of reduced vision after cataract surgery. There are a number of rarer causes of cystoid macular oedema, including several iatrogenic causes. There is sometimes a cystoid component in diabetic maculopathy. This is more common in diffuse and chronic diabetic macular oedema. Cystoid macular oedema is sometimes observed in age-related macular degeneration, particularly the retinal angiomatous proliferation subtype, although it is not the classical fluid pattern.

(f) Any one of: Fluorescein angiography, ICG angiography, OCT angiography

Feedback
Fluorescein angiography is particularly useful for investigating retinal vascular disorders. ICG (indocyanine green) angiography is useful for imaging the choroid. OCT angiography is a more recent development, and provides detailed anatomical images without the use of dyes (non-invasive technique). It is less affected by leakage, but can struggle to detect low-flow lesions, especially with turbulent flow (e.g. microaneurysms).

5. Answer

(a) Hoffer Q is likely to be more accurate for the left eye, and the axial length allows you to determine this *(1 mark for Hoffer Q; 1 mark for axial length)*

Feedback
The Hoffer Q formula has been demonstrated to be more accurate than the SRK/T formula for eyes with an axial length below 21.5 mm. Conversely the SRK/T formula was demonstrated to have better accuracy for eyes with an axial length of 27 mm or greater. As the axial length in this patient's left eye is 20.93 mm, it would be advisable to use the Hoffer Q formula to predict the correct intraocular lens implant.

(b) Axial length and average keratometry (corneal curvature or power) *(1 mark for each; either nomenclature may be used for the average keratometry)*

Feedback
Both the SRK/T and Hoffer Q formulas rely on accurate measurement of the axial length and the average keratometry. The Holladay 1 formula also relies on these two measurements. The Haigis formula additionally uses pre-operative anterior chamber depth, the Barrett Universal II formula uses 5 variables, and the

Answers: CRQs

Holladay 2 formula uses seven measurements. The Olsen formula uses ray tracing to calculate the required lens power, while the Hill-RBF method utilises artificial intelligence and machine learning to predict the best lens.

(c) Axial length, caused by corneal indentation with contact ultrasound biometry *(1 mark for axial length; 1 mark for corneal indentation)*

Feedback
Contact ultrasound biometry always produces some corneal indentation, and therefore the axial lengths recorded are shorter than those measured by immersion or optical biometry.

(d) It is not always possible to measure axial length using optical biometry

Feedback
In approximately 10% of eyes (depending on case mix) it is not possible to measure the axial length using optical biometry. This is particularly a problem with dense posterior subcapsular cataracts, although it can also be due to other media opacities or poor eye fixation. In these cases it is necessary to measure the axial length using ultrasound.

(e) 62 degrees or 242 degrees *(1 mark each)*

Feedback
The steep axis is indicated by the higher K value (in this case K2: 45.79 D at 62 degrees). Any astigmatism caused by a corneal incision at this point will reduce the steepness of this axis, and therefore reduce the total astigmatism of the eye. The steep axis will continue at 180 degrees to the higher K value (in this case 242 degrees), and the more comfortable position can be chosen. This biometry printout also has the effective negative cylinder calculated below the K values, and the steep axis will be at 90 degrees to the axis of the negative cylinder.

(f) 118.5

Feedback
As in the original SRK formula, the A-constant in the SRK/T formula has a 1:1 relationship with the intraocular lens (IOL) power. Therefore, if two lenses have the same predicted outcome the difference between the IOL powers will be the difference between the A-constants.

The biometry for the right eye gives a predicted outcome of -0.09 for a 29 dioptre SN60WF IOL.

Therefore for a lens giving the same outcome with a 28.5 dioptre IOL the A-constant must be 0.5 dioptres smaller than that of the SN60WF, therefore 118.5.

6. Answer

(a) Indocyanine green (ICG) angiography

Feedback
Image B is a slide from indocyanine green (ICG) angiography. The contrast with the fundus fluorescein angiography (FFA) image, A, is stark: rather than the diffuse

background fluorescence of FFA it is possible to see the individual choroidal vessels in addition to the vessels of the retinal circulation.

(b) Both the excitation source and fluorescence for investigation B are in the near-infrared range, with the fluorescence having a longer wavelength than the excitation source. *(1 mark each for excitation source and fluorescence, with either a statement of near-infrared or a reasonable wavelength or range given)*

Feedback
In vivo, indocyanine green (ICG) absorbs near-infrared light between approximately 790–805 nm. Its emission spectrum is also near-infrared in the range of 770–880 nm, with a peak emission of 835 nm. This is an important factor in the relative advantages of ICG over fluorescein angiography (see below).

(c) Both the excitation and fluorescence light in fluorescein angiography is absorbed and scattered by pigments in the retina and retinal pigment epithelium (including macular xanthophyll), limiting the visualisation of structures deep to these tissues. Also, fluorescein molecules rapidly extravasate from the choroidal circulation, giving rise to a diffuse background fluorescence. *(1 mark each for: scattering and absorption of excitation and fluorescence light; rapid extravasation from choroidal circulation)*

Feedback
The relatively short wavelengths of the excitation and fluorescence light in fluorescein angiography result in a greater degree of scatter and absorption by the tissues of the fundus than the near-infrared rays of indocyanine green (ICG) angiography. Indeed macular xanthophyll (mainly found in the inner and outer plexiform layers) is thought to play a physiological role in limiting damage to photoreceptors from high-energy short wavelength light. Also, as fluorescein extravasates more rapidly than ICG it quickly fills the area of the choroid with a low intensity haze that further limits the view of the choroidal circulation.

(d) Any three of:

Better visualisation through media opacities
Better visualisation of vessels behind haemorrhages
Better tolerance in photophobic patients
More accurate measurement of the size of occult choroidal neovascular membranes (CNVM)
(1 mark for each up to three marks)

Feedback
As indocyanine green (ICG) utilises light in the near-infrared spectrum the scattering from media opacities is much lower than with the shorter wavelengths used in fluorescein angiography. For a similar reason it is possible to visualise large blood vessels hidden deep to haemorrhages in the retina. As near-infrared light is barely perceptible to the human eye it is better tolerated by photophobic patients than the cobalt blue excitation light of fluorescein angiography. It is difficult to accurately measure the size of occult CNVMs with fluorescein angiography as they may be over-estimated due to leakage into neurosensory or

pigment epithelial detachments, or under-estimated due to blocked fluorescence by blood or exudate.

(e) Because indocyanine green (ICG) has a higher degree of binding to plasma proteins than fluorescein

Feedback
Indocyanine green is 98% bound to plasma proteins, with around 80% being bound to globulins (especially alpha-1-lipoproteins). Fluorescein, by comparison, is 80% protein-bound in the circulation, leaving more free molecules to extravasate. This difference is largely due to the amphiphilic nature of ICG (both hydrophilic and lipophilic) compared to the primarily hydrophilic nature of fluorescein, resulting in ICG binding to lipoproteins and phospholipids in addition to the proteins fluorescein has an affinity for.

(f) Hepatobiliary excretion

Feedback
Indocyanine green (ICG) is excreted entirely by the hepatobiliary system. Hepatic parenchymal cells take up ICG and secrete it unchanged into the bile. This typically results in discolouration of the stool for several days. Persistence of the dye in the retinal and choroidal circulation for more than 30 minutes in the late phase should raise the suspicion of reduced hepatic function.

7. Answer

(a) An X-ray tube rotates around the patient, taking a large number of X-rays from different angles, which are detected by detector plates and processed by a computer to produce the CT images. *(1 mark for describing a rotating X-ray tube and detector; 1 mark for describing processing of images by computer)*

Feedback
It is important to understand that each axial segment in a CT scan is compiled from a number of X-ray images taken at different angles which only make a useful image when put together. CT scanners use rows of small, electronic detectors rather than conventional film, so that the X-ray data can be easily compiled by the computer. CTs are acquired in the axial plane, however, the data can subsequently be reconstructed into any plane. 3D reconstructions are also possible.

(b) Opacification of the right maxillary sinus and soft tissue swelling/stranding in the right peri-orbital/facial area *(1 mark for each abnormality)*

Feedback
Sinuses are usually black on a CT scan (as they are air-filled), and subtotal opacification as seen in this image is indicative of a more radio-dense material in the sinus. This could be serous fluid, pus, haemorrhage or solid material, and the density of the material, which can be assessed on CT, can help to differentiate between these. The right peri-orbital/facial soft tissues are significantly swollen compared with the left, and there is a haziness of the subcutaneous fat (stranding) in keeping with acute inflammation.

(c) Right proptosis

Feedback
When looking at CT or MRI images you should always compare the structures on each side for asymmetry. In this scan the right globe is significantly further forwards in the orbit than the left. It is also possible to see more of the soft tissue swelling, and further opacification of the paranasal sinuses (right ethmoid sinus).

(d) Orbital cellulitis (secondary to sinusitis) *(1 mark for orbital cellulitis)*

Feedback
These features are most in keeping with an orbital cellulitis secondary to sinusitis. Bacterial spread from paranasal sinuses is the most common aetiology for orbital cellulitis.

(e) Right relative afferent pupillary defect (RAPD), which would indicate compromise of right optic nerve function *(1 mark for right RAPD; 1 mark for significance)*

Feedback
It is important to look for an RAPD whenever orbital cellulitis is suspected as this will help to differentiate blurred vision secondary to ocular surface factors from blurred vision secondary to optic nerve compromise.

(f) Any two of:

Meningitis
Cerebritis
Cavernous sinus thrombosis
Intracranial abscess
(1 mark for each correct answer; only two answers should be provided)

Feedback
Intracranial spread of infection is a potentially serious complication of orbital cellulitis. It can involve the meninges (meningitis) or brain parenchyma (cerebritis). Abscesses can form within the brain parenchyma or in the extra-axial space (e.g. subdural empyema). The inflammatory process can also cause cavernous sinus thrombosis. Complications are more likely if presentation or treatment is delayed. Thankfully with appropriate treatment these complications are rare.

Microbiology

8. Answer

(a) Fungal hyphae

Feedback
This is a slide showing fungal hyphae, which are branching filamentous structures that grow from their tips to facilitate the spread of the organism.

(b) Sabouraud agar

Feedback
Sabouraud agar is formulated to support the growth of a range of fungi. It has a relatively acidic pH to inhibit the growth of bacteria.

(c) Culturing of fungi can be slower than clinical progress

Feedback
Fungi are slow-growing in culture, and it can take up to 3 weeks to culture and identify the organism. In this time the patient's clinical condition will have progressed significantly.

(d) Acridine orange and calcofluor white *(1 mark for each)*

Feedback
Acridine orange and calcofluor white will both stain fungi and cause them to fluoresce under the appropriate lighting conditions. This can assist with the rapid identification of pathogens. A number of other stains may be used which do not require a fluorescent microscope, including Periodic Acid Schiff (PAS) and Grocott-Gömöri Methenamine Silver (GMS) stains.

(e) Any two of:

Aspergillus
Fusarium
Acremonium
(1 mark each for any two)

Feedback
Broadly speaking, it is helpful to divide fungi that can cause keratitis into filamentous fungi and yeast-like organisms. Filamentous fungi can be further subdivided into septate and non-septate organisms. Septae are visible in this slide. These septae are non-pigmented, which suggests the organism is likely to be one of *Aspergillus*, *Fusarium* or *Acremonium*.

(f) Any three of:

Contact lens wear
Corneal abrasion or trauma
Diabetes
Dry eye
Exposure to vegetable matter
Immunosuppression (e.g. steroids)
Previous corneal transplant
Reduced corneal sensation
Warm, humid environment
(1 mark for each up to a maximum of three)

Feedback
Risk factors for fungal keratitis can be divided into host factors and environmental factors. Host factors include diabetes, dry eye (e.g. Sjögren's disease), immunosuppression (e.g. systemic or topical steroids), previous corneal

transplant and reduced corneal sensation (e.g. previous herpetic disease; LASIK). Environmental factors include exposure to vegetable matter (e.g. farm workers) and warm, humid environments (e.g. travellers returning from the tropics).

Optics

9. Answer

(a) Right eye +3.00 DS/−1.50 DC axis 165°   Left eye −0.75 DS/−0.75 DC axis 5°

(1 mark for each eye)

Feedback
To convert from positive to negative cylinder, or vice versa, simply add the given sphere and cylinder power together to give the new sphere, then change the sign on the cylinder and change the axis by 90°.

(b) +2.25

Feedback
To calculate the spherical equivalent, add half of the cylinder power to the sphere power.

(c) Right cataract surgery/clear lens extraction, iseikonic lenses, contact lenses, refractive surgery *(1 mark for each, maximum 3 marks)*

Feedback
Symptomatic anisometropia following cataract surgery is commonly addressed by removing the cataract in the fellow eye (if anisometropia is predicted then second eye surgery is often prioritised).

Iseikonic lenses are a special lens form for glasses which can alter the image size to compensate for small degrees of anisometropia.

Contact lenses reduce the impact of anisometropia as relative spectacle magnification varies according to back vertex distance, which is reduced in contact lenses compared to spectacles. However, they are often poorly tolerated in the elderly.

Various forms of refractive surgery could be used to reduce or eliminate the anisometropia, although in practice it is more likely that one of the first three options would be chosen.

(d) Index myopia

Feedback
Increasing nucleosclerosis can lead to an increase in the refractive index of the lens, resulting in increasing lens power and myopic shift. Conversely this means she will require less plus (or more minus) power in her correcting lenses, resulting in decreased anisometropia. The decision on whether any treatment

at all is required at this stage will depend on whether she is symptomatic from anisometropia and/or from developing cataract in the right eye.

(e) Corneal incisions placed at 75° and/or 255°, toric intraocular lens insertion *(1 mark for each)*

Feedback
Peripheral corneal incisions can be used to reduce the corneal curvature, and therefore decrease the corneal refractive power on that axis. These can be placed as part of cataract surgery or in isolation as partial thickness incisions. Nomograms exist to predict the refractive impact depending on a number of factors, including incision length, depth and position, corneal pachymetry and patient age. Toric intraocular lenses require careful placement with respect to the angle of astigmatism, but they are unlikely to induce irregular astigmatism and can be placed through a normal phacoemulsification incision.

(f) Induced corneal astigmatism will increase with increasing distance between the limbus and the incision

Feedback
There is a risk of irregular astigmatism and glare if an incision is placed too near the centre of the optical zone.

10. Answer

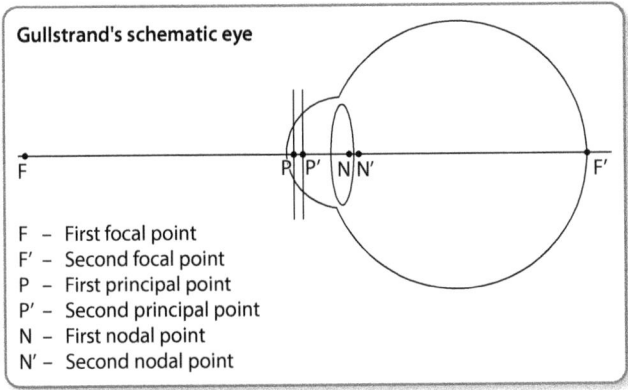

Gullstrand's schematic eye

F — First focal point
F' — Second focal point
P — First principal point
P' — Second principal point
N — First nodal point
N' — Second nodal point

(a) *(1 mark for each correctly labelled point)*

Feedback
Gullstrand's schematic eye relies on describing the optical system of the eye in terms of cardinal points. Light originating from the first focal point will be refracted into parallel rays by the optical system, whereas parallel light entering the optical system will be focused at the second focal point (which lies on the retina in the schematic eye as it represents emmetropia). The first and second principal points lie close together in the anterior chamber, where the principal planes meet the principal axis. The first nodal point lies immediately anterior to

the posterior pole of the lens, whereas the second nodal point lies in the vitreous just behind the posterior pole of the lens.

(b) The nodal point in the reduced schematic eye lies in the posterior lens material

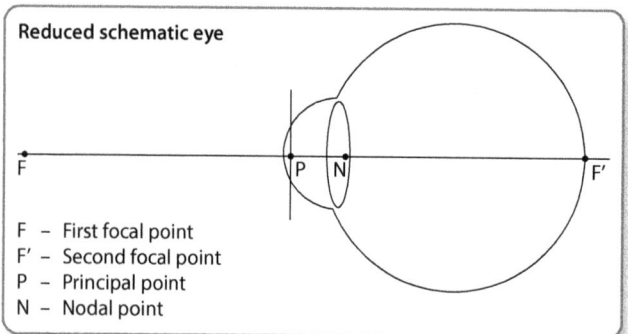

Reduced schematic eye

F - First focal point
F' - Second focal point
P - Principal point
N - Nodal point

Feedback
The reduced schematic eye uses a single principal point and a single nodal point to create a further simplified schematic representation of refraction in the eye. It essentially treats the eye as a single refracting surface with a power of +58.6 dioptres.

(c) The refractive power at an interface between two media is dependent on the difference in refractive index between the two media rather than the absolute refractive index. The cornea and tear film has an interface with the air, which has a refractive index of 1 compared to the cornea's refractive index of 1.37. The refractive index of the aqueous is 1.33, and the vitreous approximately 1.34, compared to the crystalline lens which varies from 1.38–1.42. Therefore, there is a greater refractive effect at the air-cornea interface than at either the aqueous-lens or lens–vitreous interfaces (*2 marks*). Furthermore the radius of curvature of the cornea is smaller than that of the lens, and as the power of a refractive surface is inversely proportional to the radius of curvature this is also a factor in the greater contribution of the cornea to the total refractive power of the eye (*1 mark*).

11. Answer

(a) The accommodative convergence/accommodation (AC/A) ratio is the number of prism dioptres of convergence (*1 mark*) induced by each dioptre of accommodation (*1 mark*)

Feedback
The AC/A ratio is generally a fixed relationship for each individual that stays constant from childhood to presbyopia.

(b) The normal range is 3:1 to 5:1

Feedback
This means that for each dioptre of accommodation, there is normally 3 to 5 prism dioptres of accommodative convergence.

The AC/A ratio can be temporarily offset by glasses or drugs that reduce the amount of accommodation needed, and permanently changed by strabismus surgery. Thus, there are optical, pharmacological and surgical management strategies for managing accommodative strabismus.

(c) The AC/A ratio is 9.5:1 *(2 marks)*

$$AC/A = IPD\,(cm) + \frac{(Near\,PCT) - (Distance\,PCT)}{Near\,fixation\,distance\,in\,dioptres}$$

$$= 5.5 + \frac{(+8) - (-4)}{3}$$

$$= 5.5 + 4$$

$$= 9.5$$

(IPD: interpupillary distance; PCT: prism cover test)

Feedback
An alternative way of expressing the heterophoria method formula is:

AC/A = IPD + (near fixation distance in m) (near PCT − distance PCT)

This uses 0.33 m, instead of 3 D, as the near fixation measurement.

Remember that when expressing the size of the deviation (as PCT), this has a positive sign for esodeviations, and a negative sign for exodeviations. For example, a 4 Δ esophoria should be used as +4 in the AC/A calculation, whereas a 6 Δ exotropia is expressed as −6.

The gradient method is an alternative way of calculating the AC/A ratio. Whereas the heterophoria method uses the change in deviation for near versus distance, the gradient method takes measurements at the same distance, but induces changes in accommodation with different lenses. The IPD is not needed for the gradient method. Typically the calculated AC/A ratio is lower with the gradient method than with the heterophoria method.

(d) This will dramatically reduce or eliminate the esotropia *(1 mark)*. This patient has a 30 Δ esotropia without glasses. As the AC/A ratio is 6:1, each dioptre of accommodation results in 6 Δ of convergence. Prescribing the full hypermetropic glasses correction will reduce the amount of accommodation needed by 5 dioptres *(1 mark)*, which will therefore reduce the amount of convergence by:

$$6 \times 5 = 30\,\Delta\,(1\,mark)$$

In theory, therefore, this should eliminate the patient's esotropia.

Feedback
This child has a fully accommodative (refractive) esotropia. This occurs in significantly hypermetropic children and the deviation is by definition eliminated by glasses wear. Taking the glasses off will result in the squint recurring. The treatment is full-time glasses wear.

If the esotropia is reduced but not eliminated by the hypermetropic correction, this is known as a partially accommodative esotropia and may require squint surgery in addition to glasses wear.

12. Answer

(a) Goldmann applanation tonometer

(b) At the tip of the tonometer head, two prisms are placed with their bases in opposite directions.

This is to split the operator's view of the fluorescein-stained tear meniscus, which is formed by the contact between the tonometer head and the cornea (*1 mark*).

This allows precise adjustment of the force on the dial, until the area of contact is seen to be correct (corresponding to a circle 3.06 mm in diameter) by adjustment of the mires. It is only when the area of contact is correct that the force applied is proportional to the intraocular pressure (*1 mark*).

(c) Applanation tonometry is based on the Imbert–Fick principle:

$$P = \frac{F}{A}$$

where P is the pressure, F is the force of application and A is the area of applanation.

The force of application is directly proportional to the intraocular pressure (IOP) when the area of contact is a circle whose diameter is exactly 3.06 mm. At this area of contact, the repulsive effect of corneal rigidity and attractive effect of the surface tension of the tear meniscus are balanced. The force is increased until the mires are aligned at their inner margins, indicating that the area of corneal contact is correct. At this point, the reading on the dial is multiplied by 10 to give the IOP in mmHg.

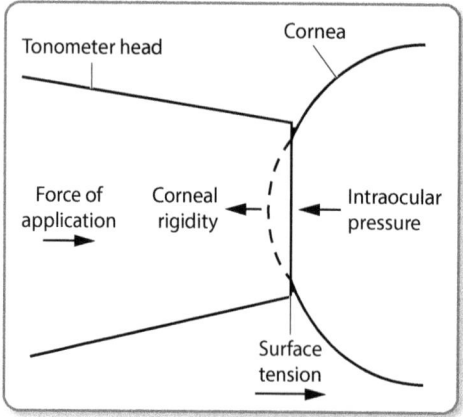

(1 mark for Imbert–Fick principle with equation, 3 marks for forces correctly illustrated on an appropriate diagram: force of application against intraocular pressure: 1 mark, corneal rigidity: 1 mark, surface tension: 1 mark)

(d) 1

Feedback
In order to ensure the correct area of contact between the tonometer head and the cornea, the applanation force (force of application) must be adjusted until the mires are aligned at their inner margins.

In part 1, the applanation force applied is too low, and the current reading will be lower than the true IOP. In part 2, the mires are aligned correctly and the IOP measurement can be taken. The configuration in part 3 is not seen due to the prisms splitting the view of the mires. In part 4, the applanation force applied is too high, and the current reading will be higher than the true IOP.

(e) Any two of:

Corneal thickness (thicker or thinner than average)
Excessive or inadequate fluorescein
High astigmatism
Pressure on the globe whilst holding the lids open
Patient 'squeezing' or blepharospasm
Breath holding (Valsalva)
Patient wearing a tight collar
Failure to calibrate the tonometer
Incorrect eyepiece on slit lamp
Other force interfering with the tonometer arm (e.g. face mask)
(½ mark each)

Feedback
Care should be taken to avoid sources of error with Goldmann tonometry, as all of these factors may lead to under- or overestimation of the true intraocular pressure. Many of these are avoided with proper technique.

For example, holding the lids open should be done with pressure on the bony orbit and not on the globe; adequate explanation and topical anaesthesia can help to maximise patient comfort and minimise 'squeezing' of the lids.

In patients with a high degree of regular corneal astigmatism (e.g. >3 dioptres), the measurement should ideally be taken at 43° to the axis of the minus cylinder: if the prism is marked with degrees, line up the axis of the minus cylinder with the red line on the prism holder.

Corneal pachymetry should be performed to help interpretation of the results.

(f) Due to the above-average corneal thickness, the measured intraocular pressure (IOP) is likely to be an overestimate of the true IOP

Feedback

The accuracy of applanation tonometry relies on the central corneal thickness being within the normal range. The mean central corneal thickness in the general population is approximately 550 μm. This patient has significantly thicker than average corneas, meaning that the measured IOP is likely to overestimate the true IOP.

Whilst it is essential to know the corneal thickness to aid interpretation of the IOP result, the use of specific correction algorithms or nomograms to then adjust the IOP result is controversial. What is not controversial is that corneal thickness should be taken into account in management decisions, with thin corneas being an independent risk factor for glaucomatous progression.

Chapter 2

Exam Paper 2: Structured Practice Paper

Questions: SBAs

120 SBAs to be answered in 3 hours

For each question, please select the single best answer.

Anatomy

1. Regarding the maxillary sinus, which of the following statements is false?
   A It is lined by mucoperiosteum with pseudostratified columnar ciliated epithelium
   B It opens into the inferior meatus through the hiatus semilunaris
   C Its roof contains the infraorbital nerve and blood vessels
   D Maxillary sinusitis can result in dental pain

2. Regarding orbital fractures, which of the following statements is false?
   A Blowout fractures of the orbit typically present with diplopia and exophthalmos
   B Little force is required to fracture the medial wall of the orbit
   C Numbness of the cheek suggests trigeminal nerve damage
   D Patients with orbital fractures should avoid blowing their nose

3. Which of the following structures pass through the inferior orbital fissure?
   A Branches of the pterygopalatine ganglion
   B Infraorbital vein
   C Zygomatic nerve
   D All of the above

4. Regarding the eyebrows, which of the following statements is incorrect?
   A   The arterial supply is from the supraorbital and supratrochlear arteries
   B   The eyebrows are drawn medially by contraction of the corrugator supercilii muscle, which is supplied by the fifth cranial nerve
   C   The eyebrows are raised by contraction of the frontalis muscle, which is supplied by the seventh cranial nerve
   D   The venous drainage is into the facial vein via the angular vein

5. Regarding the eyelids, which of the following statements is true?
   A   Orbital cellulitis refers to post-septal infection
   B   The lacrimal sac lies posterior to the orbital septum
   C   The tarsal plate of the upper lid is 5 mm in height
   D   There are approximately 50 eyelashes in the upper lid and 25 in the lower lid

6. Where is the origin of the inferior oblique muscle?
   A   Body of the sphenoid
   B   Common tendinous ring
   C   Fascial sheath of inferior rectus
   D   Orbital floor

7. In the extraocular muscles, what is the approximate innervation ratio of motor neurons to muscle fibres?
   A   1:2 to 1:7
   B   1:50 to 1:100
   C   1: 300 to 1:600
   D   1:1,000 to 1:2,000

8. Optic chiasmal lesions are associated with characteristic visual field defects. Which of the following is an incorrect association between lesion and field defect?
   A   Craniopharyngioma: superior bitemporal field defect
   B   Olfactory groove meningioma: inferior bitemporal field defect
   C   Pituitary adenoma: superior bitemporal field defect
   D   Sphenoid wing meningioma: junctional scotoma

9. Which of the following best describes the location of the accessory lacrimal glands of Krause?
   A   Anterior to the grey line adjacent to the lashes
   B   Around the conjunctival fornix
   C   At the border of the tarsal plate
   D   In the subtarsal sulcus

10. Which of the following is a branch of the external carotid artery?

    A   Inferior thyroid artery
    B   Mandibular artery
    C   Posterior auricular artery
    D   Posterior ciliary artery

11. A patient has a left-sided inferior rectus, inferior oblique and medial rectus weakness with a bilateral ptosis and right superior rectus underaction. Where is the lesion located?

    A   Cavernous sinus
    B   Edinger–Westphal nucleus
    C   Left third nerve fascicle
    D   Left third nerve nucleus

12. Which of the following rectus muscles usually only receives blood from a single anterior ciliary artery?

    A   Inferior rectus
    B   Lateral rectus
    C   Medial rectus
    D   Superior rectus

13. Which of the following statements about the retinal blood supply is false?

    A   A blood–tissue barrier is created for the retina by the action of tight junctions and regulated membrane transport proteins
    B   The choroidal circulation has a flow rate of ~150 mm/s whereas the retinal circulation has a flow rate of ~25 mm/s
    C   The inner third of the retina is supplied by branches of the central retinal artery whereas the outer two-thirds is supplied by the choroidal circulation
    D   The retina consumes more oxygen per unit weight than any other tissue

14. Wieger's ligament connects which two structures?

    A   Anterior hyaloid face and ciliary body
    B   Anterior hyaloid face and posterior lens capsule
    C   Posterior hyaloid face and fovea
    D   Posterior hyaloid face and optic nerve

15. What is the normal length of the horizontal component of the lacrimal canaliculi between the ampulla and common canaliculus?

    A   4–6 mm
    B   8–10 mm
    C   12–14 mm
    D   16–18 mm

16. Which of the following statements about the sclera is false?

    A Pigmented spots may be seen on the episclera where melanocytes have migrated through the emissary canals
    B The lamina fusca lies immediately superficial to the scleral stroma
    C The sclera is covered by the fascia bulbi, separating it from the orbital fat
    D The sclera is thinnest behind the insertions of the extraocular muscles

17. Which of the following bones does not contribute to the boundaries of the pterygopalatine fossa?

    A Ethmoid
    B Maxilla
    C Palatine
    D Sphenoid

18. Which vessel does the left common carotid artery most commonly arise from?

    A Aortic arch
    B Brachiocephalic trunk
    C Costocervical trunk
    D Subclavian artery

19. Which of the following statements about the epithelium of the ciliary body is true?

    A The basement membrane of the pigmented ciliary epithelium is continuous with the internal limiting membrane of the retina
    B The bases of the inner ciliary epithelial cells face the apices of the outer ciliary epithelial cells
    C The inner pigmented ciliary epithelium is continuous anteriorly with the pigmented posterior epithelium of the iris
    D The transition between the neuroretina and the non-pigmented ciliary epithelium occurs at the ora serrata

20. In an eye with no previous history of intraocular surgery, where is the most common site of globe rupture following blunt trauma?

    A Inferomedial quadrant
    B Insertion of the recti
    C Peripheral cornea
    D Posterior to the equator

21. What is the normal fluid volume of the anterior chamber?

    A 250 μL
    B 375 μL
    C 500 μL
    D 625 μL

22. In the absence of pathology, in which layer of the choroid do blood vessels leak fluorescein dye?

    A   Bruch's membrane
    B   Choriocapillaris
    C   Haller's layer
    D   Sattler's layer

Biochemistry

23. Which of the following cell types does not contain mitochondria?

    A   Erythrocyte
    B   Lymphocyte
    C   Ovum
    D   Sperm

24. What is the principal type of glucose metabolism in the lens?

    A   Aerobic glycolysis
    B   Anaerobic glycolysis
    C   Pentose phosphate pathway
    D   Sorbitol pathway

25. Regarding the role of different matrix metalloproteinases (MMPs) in the cornea, which of the following statements is false?

    A   MMP-2 helps to maintain the normal framework of the cornea
    B   MMP-2 is primarily involved in forming new extracellular matrix
    C   MMP-9 is involved in corneal epithelial remodelling
    D   MMPs include gelatinases and collagenases

26. Which type of intercellular junction is found at the apex of the retinal pigment epithelial cells?

    A   Adherens junctions
    B   Belt desmosomes
    C   Gap junctions
    D   Tight junctions

27. Which of the following does not contain significant quantities of fibrillin?

    A   The aqueous
    B   The lens capsule
    C   The vitreous
    D   The zonules

28. Which of the following statements about enzyme-linked immunosorbent assay (ELISA) is false?

    A It can be used to quantify hormones
    B It can detect antigens or antibodies even when only present in small quantities
    C It is used as a test for HIV
    D It utilises radioisotopes to label test targets

29. Regarding the human visual cycle, which of the following statements is true?

    A 11-*cis* retinal is an isoform of vitamin C
    B Chromophore regeneration occurs in the retinal pigment epithelium
    C Photon absorption induces photoisomerisation of all-*trans* retinal to 11-*cis* retinal
    D Retinal is bound to opsins by hydrogen bonds

30. What is the major neurotransmitter at the synapse between photoreceptors and bipolar cells?

    A Acetylcholine
    B GABA
    C Glutamate
    D Noradrenaline

31. Which of the following is a property of actin?

    A It is a microtubule
    B It is an intermediate filament
    C It is 40 nm in diameter
    D It is flexible

Embryology, growth and development

32. Which of the following sequences is the correct morphological progression?

    A Morula; blastocyst; zygote
    B Morula; zygote; blastocyst
    C Zygote; blastocyst; morula
    D Zygote; morula; blastocyst

33. Which of the following muscles is not formed by the second pharyngeal arch?

    A Corrugator supercilii
    B Stapedius
    C Stylohyoid
    D Temporalis

34. Which of the following structures is not derived from mesoderm?

    A The endothelium of Schlemm's canal
    B The endothelium of the tunica vasculosa lentis
    C The epithelium of the cornea
    D The extraocular muscles

35. Which one of the following statements about paranasal sinus development is false?

    A The ethmoid sinuses are normally present at birth
    B The frontal sinuses are usually absent at birth
    C The maxillary sinuses are the first sinuses to appear
    D The sphenoid sinus normally appears two months after birth

36. At what stage of gestation does the hyaloid artery disappear?

    A 16 weeks
    B 20 weeks
    C 24 weeks
    D 34 weeks

Genetics

37. Which of the following corneal dystrophies is inherited in an autosomal recessive pattern?

    A Granular dystrophy
    B Lattice dystrophy
    C Macular dystrophy
    D Reis–Buckler dystrophy

38. Which of the following is the correct sequence of phases of mitosis?

    A Interphase; prophase; anaphase; metaphase; telophase
    B Interphase; prophase; metaphase; anaphase; telophase
    C Prophase; interphase; anaphase; metaphase; telophase
    D Prophase; interphase; metaphase; anaphase; telophase

39. Which of the following statements regarding congenital aniridia is false?

    A Autosomal dominant is the most common mode of inheritance
    B It is associated with nephroblastoma (Wilms' tumour) in 90% of patients
    C It can be associated with urogenital malformations and intellectual disability
    D *PAX6* variants on chromosome 11 are the most common cause of aniridia

40. Regarding the polymerase chain reaction (PCR), which of the following statements is true?

   A   30 cycles results in 10^{30} copies of the target DNA
   B   It involves denaturing the DNA
   C   Synthesis occurs in the 3' to 5' direction
   D   This process requires an RNA polymerase enzyme

41. Regarding human chromosomes, which of the following statements is false?

   A   Chromosome 6 is bigger than chromosome 13
   B   Giemsa staining produces contrasting bands on chromosomes
   C   Inversions can disrupt the segregation of chromosomes during meiosis
   D   Translocation usually results in loss of DNA

42. You are studying gene frequencies in a population with regard to a specific single-gene disorder. In which of the following circumstances does the Hardy–Weinberg equilibrium still apply?

   A   Mating between first cousins
   B   Mutations affecting the gene in question
   C   Natural selection
   D   X-linked conditions

43. In the presence of irreparable damage to a cell's DNA, what process will p53 initiate?

   A   Apoptosis
   B   Meiosis
   C   Mitosis
   D   Necrosis

44. Which of the following ocular conditions is not associated with Down syndrome?

   A   Brushfield spots
   B   Cataract
   C   Coloboma
   D   Keratoconus

45. What is the cardinal ocular feature of Von Hippel–Lindau syndrome?

   A   Cerebellar haemangioblastoma
   B   Optic nerve glioma
   C   Retinal angiomata
   D   Retinal hamartomas

46. Which term describes chromosomes with the centromere located at the centre of the chromosome?

    A Acrocentric
    B Holocentric
    C Metacentric
    D Telocentric

Immunology

47. Regarding the complement system, which of the following statements is incorrect?

    A Extrahepatic synthesis of complement proteins occurs in macrophages
    B Regulatory mechanisms preventing inappropriate complement activation include factor B
    C The alternative complement pathway is initiated by direct binding of C3b to the surface of an organism
    D The complement system is an enzyme cascade

48. Regarding cell death in immune reactions, which of the following statements is false?

    A CD8$^+$ glycoproteins are found on the surface of cytotoxic T cells
    B Cytotoxic T cells release perforin which contributes to cell lysis
    C Killing of cells by NK cells involves necrosis induced by granzymes
    D The complement cascade results in cell death by osmotic lysis

49. Regarding major histocompatibility complex (MHC) class II molecules, which of the following statements is false?

    A Antigen presenting cells are the only cells that express these constitutively in high levels
    B MHC class II molecules can be expressed by some epithelial cells
    C The peptides they are complexed with are recognised by CD4$^+$ T helper cells
    D They present predominantly intracellular antigens that have been degraded in endosomes

50. Which of the following factors contributes least to the generation of antibody diversity?

    A Germline mutations
    B Junctional diversification
    C Multiple gene segments contributing to heavy and light chains
    D Somatic mutations

Investigations and imaging

51. Which of the following statements regarding the visual-evoked potential (VEP) is incorrect?

    A Abnormal chiasmal crossing is seen in albinism
    B Flash VEP requires the patient to be conscious
    C VEP is essentially a limited electroencephalogram (EEG)
    D VEP is tested in response to a changing visual stimulus

Microbiology

52. Which of the following tests indicates full immunity to hepatitis B if positive?

    A Hepatitis B core antibody (HBcAb) IgG
    B Hepatitis B core antibody (HBcAb) IgM
    C Hepatitis B envelope antibody (HBeAb) IgG
    D Hepatitis B surface antibody (HBsAb) IgG

53. Which one of the following is a DNA virus?

    A Adenovirus
    B Coxsackie
    C Influenza A
    D Measles

54. Which one of the following bacterial enzymes allows bacteria to resist phagocytosis?

    A Coagulase
    B Collagenase
    C Hyaluronidase
    D Streptokinase

55. Regarding viral inclusion bodies, which of the following statements is false?

    A Cowdry type A inclusion bodies can be seen in varicella zoster infection
    B Haematoxylin and eosin (H&E) staining is useful for visualising inclusion bodies
    C Inclusion bodies can be seen in both the cytoplasm and the nucleus
    D Owl's eye inclusion bodies are suggestive of herpes simplex virus

56. The following antibiotics interfere with bacterial protein synthesis. Which antibiotic does not target the 50S subunit of the bacterial ribosome?

    A Chloramphenicol
    B Clarithromycin

C Clindamycin
D Gentamicin

57. Which of the following statements about bacterial cell walls is false?
    A Beta-lactam antibiotics interfere with bacterial cell wall synthesis
    B Gram negative bacteria are protected by an outer membrane composed of glycosaminoglycans
    C Peptidoglycans are a key structural component of bacterial cell walls
    D The cell walls of Gram positive bacteria are generally thicker than those of Gram negative bacteria

58. Which of the following most accurately describes endotoxins?
    A They activate the alternative complement pathway
    B They are highly antigenic
    C They are proteins released during cell lysis
    D They do not lead to a systemic inflammatory response

59. Which of the following risk factors is most commonly implicated in microbial keratitis?
    A Contact lens wear
    B Diabetes
    C Dry eyes
    D Removal of a corneal suture

60. Which of the following is not true of *Acanthamoeba*?
    A *Acanthamoeba* are found in soil
    B *Acanthamoeba* are single-celled, eukaryotic organisms
    C Chlorination of water kills *Acanthamoeba* cysts
    D Trophozoites produce enzymes which aid tissue penetration

61. Which of the following statements regarding toxocara is true?
    A An IgE-mediated immune response will be mounted
    B Cysts are transmitted via canine or feline faeces
    C It is typically bilateral
    D Systemic infection is usually fatal

Optics

62. Which of the following prisms causes 180° deviation with no left-to-right transposition?
    A Dove prism
    B Fresnel prism

C   Porro prism
D   Wollaston prism

63. Which of the following transpositions is incorrect?

    A   +4.50/−2.25 × 140° = +2.25/+2.25 × 50°
    B   −3.75/−1.75 × 80° = −4.50/+1.75 × 170°
    C   +2.00/−3.25 × 20° = −1.25/+3.25 × 110°
    D   −1.75/−1.25 × 60° = −3.00/+1.25 × 150°

64. Which value is not required in the SRK formula for intraocular lens calculation?

    A   A-constant for the desired intraocular lens
    B   Anterior chamber depth
    C   Average keratometry reading
    D   Axial length

65. Which of the following Volk examination lenses has an image magnification factor of 0.93?

    A   60 dioptre
    B   66 dioptre
    C   78 dioptre
    D   90 dioptre

66. What is the radius of curvature (in mm) of the anterior surface of the cornea in the Gullstrand schematic eye?

    A   5.7
    B   6.8
    C   7.0
    D   7.7

67. What is the dioptric lens power of a simple magnifying glass (loupe) with a magnification of 2.5×?

    A   2.5
    B   4
    C   10
    D   25

68. An object lies between the centre of curvature and the principal focus of a concave mirror. How is the image formed by the mirror best described?

    A   Real, inverted, diminished
    B   Real, inverted, enlarged
    C   Virtual, erect, diminished
    D   Virtual, erect, enlarged

69. Which of the following statements regarding vergence is false?

   A A concave lens of second focal length −50 cm has a power of −2 dioptres
   B A convex lens of +90 dioptres has a second focal length of 1.11 cm
   C The first and second focal lengths of a contact lens are equal
   D The power of a lens increases as its second focal length decreases

70. What is the refractive index of the cornea?

   A 1.31
   B 1.37
   C 1.40
   D 1.52

71. How is surface illumination related to the distance from the light source?

   A Directly proportional
   B Directly proportional to the square root
   C Inversely proportional
   D Inversely proportional to the square

72. Regarding stereoacuity, which of the following statements is incorrect?

   A A stereoacuity of 3,000 seconds of arc or better excludes significant amblyopia
   B Bilateral, simultaneous stimulation of the retina occurs within Panum's fusional area
   C The Titmus (Wirt fly) stereo test requires polarising glasses
   D The TNO stereo test requires red-green filter glasses

73. What is the average dioptric power of an aphakic eye?

   A 19
   B 22
   C 43
   D 58

74. Which of the following statements about lasers is false?

   A An infrared filter in the eyepiece of the Nd:YAG laser allows the laser output to be seen as a red dot to facilitate aiming
   B Argon blue light is not recommended for macular lesions because of absorption by xanthophyll
   C The distance between the reflectors at either end of the gain medium is a multiple of the wavelength of the laser
   D The Nd:YAG laser has a wavelength of 1,064 nm

75. What is the accommodative power required for a myope with a −1.5 dioptre prescription to read unaided at 25 cm?

   A 1 dioptre
   B 2.5 dioptres
   C 5.5 dioptres
   D 7 dioptres

76. Which Purkinje–Sanson image is inverted?

   A Image I
   B Image II
   C Image III
   D Image IV

77. Which of the following adaptations of the eye does not reduce spherical aberration at the retina?

   A Graduated corneal curvature
   B Iris position
   C Variable refractive index within the lens
   D Vitreous at the posterior lens surface acting as a doublet lens

78. Which one of the following statements about the Hruby lens is incorrect?

   A It has a power of −58.6 dioptres
   B It is used with its concave surface towards the observer
   C The retinal image formed is virtual, erect and diminished
   D The retinal image formed lies within the eye of the patient

79. Which of the following prescriptions is an example of 'with the rule' astigmatism?

   A −5.25 DS/ +2.50 DC axis 180°
   B −1.50 DS/ −1.00 DC axis 45°
   C +3.00 DS/ +2.25 DC axis 85°
   D +3.50 DS/ −0.75 DC axis 90°

80. What visual angle is subtended by a letter on the 6/6 line of a Snellen chart at 6 m?

   A 1 minute of arc
   B 1 second of arc
   C 5 minutes of arc
   D 5 seconds of arc

81. What is the lens to object working distance of a simple magnifying glass of 2.5 × magnification?

    A   2.5 cm
    B   5 cm
    C   10 cm
    D   25 cm

82. The image produced by a convex lens is erect, virtual and at infinity. Where is the object located?

    A   At the first principal focus
    B   At the second principal focus
    C   Between the first principal focus and the lens
    D   Between the second principal focus and the lens

83. Which of the following is not a factor that determines the angle of deviation of a triangular prism?

    A   Angle of incidence of the light ray
    B   Refracting angle of the prism
    C   Refractive index of the prism material
    D   Width of prism base

Pathology

84. Flexner-Wintersteiner rosettes are a characteristic histopathological finding in which tumour?

    A   Capillary haemangioma
    B   Choroidal melanoma
    C   Optic nerve glioma
    D   Retinoblastoma

85. Which of the following describes glaucoma secondary to outflow obstruction by engorged macrophages following leakage of lens protein through an intact capsule into the anterior chamber?

    A   Phacoanaphylactic glaucoma
    B   Phacolytic glaucoma
    C   Phacomorphic glaucoma
    D   Lens particle glaucoma

86. Which of the following statements about keratoconus is false?

    A   Down syndrome is a risk factor for keratoconus
    B   Eye rubbing is a risk factor for progression
    C   Iron deposition at the base of the cone may be seen as a Fleischer ring
    D   Progression is generally most rapid in the fifth decade of life

87. Which one of the following does not characteristically give rise to a granulomatous reaction?

    A   Behçet's disease
    B   Chalazion
    C   Lyme disease
    D   Syphilis

88. Which one of the following tumours is malignant?

    A   Adenoma
    B   Fibrosarcoma
    C   Leiomyoma
    D   Neurofibroma

89. Where in the retina are cotton wool spots found?

    A   Bruch's membrane
    B   Nerve fibre layer
    C   Outer plexiform layer
    D   Between the photoreceptors and the RPE

90. Which of the following is not a poor prognostic factor in choroidal melanoma?

    A   Duplication of 8q
    B   Epithelioid cell type
    C   Monosomy 3
    D   Spindle cell type

91. Pathophysiological changes following retinal detachment include all of the following apart from:

    A   Degeneration of photoreceptors
    B   Proliferation and migration of the retinal pigment epithelium
    C   Subretinal lipid exudation
    D   Subretinal recruitment of macrophages

92. A 62-year-old woman is admitted to the ophthalmology ward with suspected corneal graft rejection. Which of the following is the most significant risk factor for graft rejection?

    A   Keratoconus
    B   Loose sutures

C Older age
D Small grafts

93. A young woman attends eye casualty having sustained an injury to the right eye from a golf ball. Which of the following is most likely to lead to an early rise in intraocular pressure?

   A Angle recession
   B Large hyphaema
   C Peripheral anterior synechiae formation
   D Vitreous haemorrhage

Pharmacology

94. Regarding G-protein-coupled receptors, which of the following statements is false?

   A G proteins catalyse the conversion of GTP to GDP
   B The nicotinic acetylcholine receptor is an example of this type of receptor
   C They are coupled to intracellular effector systems via G proteins
   D They contain seven transmembrane domains

95. Regarding competitive antagonists, which of the following statements is true?

   A Brimonidine is an example of a competitive antagonist at the α_2 adrenoceptor
   B In the presence of a competitive antagonist, the agonist logarithmic dose-response curve is shifted to the right
   C In the presence of a partial agonist, they activate the receptor
   D They reduce the maximum possible response elicited by the agonist

96. Which one of the following drugs increases the risk of intraoperative floppy iris syndrome during cataract surgery?

   A Atropine
   B Fluoxetine
   C Tamsulosin
   D Tricyclic antidepressants

97. Regarding topical ophthalmic medication, which of the following statements is false?

   A Excess lacrimation reduces trans-corneal drug absorption
   B The corneal stroma is hydrophilic
   C The principal barrier to intraocular penetration is the corneal endothelium
   D The volume of a typical drop exceeds the capacity of the conjunctival sac

98. Which of the following medications does not risk the systemic side effects of dry mouth, tachycardia and urinary retention?

   A   Atropine
   B   Cyclopentolate
   C   Ipratropium
   D   Pyridostigmine

99. Which of the following is not a systemic effect of glucocorticoid corticosteroids?

   A   An increase in gluconeogenesis
   B   Decreased fibroblast function
   C   Increased osteoblast function
   D   Increased protein breakdown

100. What is the pharmacological action of edrophonium in the Tensilon test?

   A   Acetylcholinesterase inhibition
   B   Acetylcholinesterase potentiation
   C   Direct acetylcholine receptor agonist
   D   Direct acetylcholine receptor antagonist

101. Which of the following is associated with mitomycin-C?

   A   DNA crosslinking
   B   Only effective at certain points in the cell cycle
   C   Significant toxicity to the corneal epithelium
   D   Use during cataract surgery to reduce scarring

102. Regarding the monitoring of anticoagulants, which of the following statements is correct?

   A   Intravenous unfractionated heparin does not require routine monitoring, but can be monitored using the activated partial thromboplastin time if required
   B   Low molecular weight heparins do not require routine monitoring, but can be monitored using anti-Xa levels if required
   C   The international normalised ratio is a ratio of the sample thromboplastin time to a standard
   D   Warfarin should ideally be monitored more frequently during the first trimester of pregnancy

103. Which one of the following substances will not produce mydriasis?

   A   Amphetamine
   B   Cocaine
   C   Heroin
   D   MDMA

Physiology

104. What is the approximate maximal spectral sensitivity of rod photoreceptors (in nanometres)?

    A   400
    B   460
    C   500
    D   560

105. Regarding colour vision defects, which of the following statements is true?

    A   Deuteranopia occurs in 5% of men
    B   Dichromatism results in a reduced range of colour detection
    C   The gene for blue (short wavelength) cone pigment is on chromosome 11
    D   Tritanomaly is characterised by the absence of blue cone function

106. Which of these statements is true regarding the pituitary gland?

    A   Follicle-stimulating hormone is produced by the posterior pituitary
    B   Glucocorticoids exert positive feedback on the hypothalamus
    C   Pituitary adenomas always result in either over- or under-secretion of hormones
    D   Somatomedins, e.g. IGF-1, result in decreased secretion of growth hormone

107. Which of the following nerves forms the afferent limb of the oculocardiac reflex?

    A   Optic nerve (II)
    B   Oculomotor nerve (III)
    C   Trigeminal nerve (V)
    D   Vagus nerve (X)

108. Which of the following does not occur when the ciliary muscle contracts?

    A   Aqueous outflow increases
    B   Axial length increases and equatorial diameter decreases
    C   The choroid is pulled anteriorly
    D   The tension on the zonules increases

109. Regarding vitamin B12 deficiency, which of the following statements is incorrect?

    A   It can cause a painless, bilateral optic neuropathy that may precede anaemia
    B   Homocysteine levels may be elevated
    C   The most common reason is inadequate dietary intake
    D   Vitamin B12 is a cofactor required by methionine synthase

110. Which of the following statements regarding osmolality is incorrect?
    A If a salt dissociates entirely into two ions in solution, 1 mole of the salt will give rise to 2 osmoles
    B Osmolality refers to osmoles per litre of solution
    C Osmoreceptors are found outside the blood–brain barrier
    D Plasma has an osmolality of approximately 280–305 mosmol/kg

111. Which of the following statements about lacrimal gland secretions is false?
    A Lactoferrin is present in significant quantities
    B Lysozyme in tears has an antibacterial role
    C The principal secretory immunoglobulin in tears is IgG
    D The tears are approximately isotonic with serum

112. Which one of the following is responsible for producing the mucin layer of the ocular tear film?
    A Conjunctival goblet cells
    B Glands of Wolfring
    C Krause's glands
    D Meibomian glands

113. What is the approximate water content of vitreous humour?
    A 60%
    B 75%
    C 85%
    D 99%

114. Regarding aqueous outflow, which of the following statements is true?
    A Aqueous drained via the trabecular route passes into the choroidal circulation
    B The innermost portion of the trabecular meshwork has the highest resistance
    C Uveoscleral outflow contributes 2–3% of aqueous outflow
    D Uveoscleral outflow is largely independent of intraocular pressure

115. Which of the following statements about the optic radiations is true?
    A Fibres corresponding to the peripheral retina have a more direct course than those corresponding to the macula
    B Meyer's loop passes anteriorly around the frontal horn of the lateral ventricle
    C The cell bodies of the nerve fibres are found in the lateral geniculate nucleus
    D The parietal optic radiation carries information from the inferior retina

116. Which statement about cerebrospinal fluid (CSF) composition under physiological conditions is false?

   A CSF has a lower chloride concentration than plasma
   B CSF has a lower glucose concentration than plasma
   C CSF has a higher magnesium concentration than plasma
   D CSF pH is lower than that of plasma

117. Which of the following statements about the magnocellular and parvocellular pathways is incorrect?

   A Magnocellular ganglions project to layers 1 and 2 in the lateral geniculate nucleus
   B Parvocellular ganglions are predominantly found in the peripheral retina
   C The parvocellular pathway is colour sensitive but has lower contrast sensitivity than the magnocellular pathway
   D The parvocellular pathway terminates primarily in layer 4Cβ in the primary visual cortex

Statistics and evidence-based medicine

118. A study investigates whether a new treatment can reduce the risk of blindness in a given population. 50 patients received the new treatment, of whom 5 went blind during the study period. 100 patients received a placebo, of whom 20 went blind during the study period. What is the absolute risk reduction of this treatment compared to placebo?

   A 10%
   B 15%
   C 50%
   D 75%

119. What is the highest phase of clinical trial that a drug must go through in order to be granted a marketing licence?

   A I
   B II
   C III
   D IV

120. Which of the following statistical tests does not typically assume normal distribution of the sample?

   A Analysis of variance
   B χ^2
   C Pearson's test
   D Student's t test

Questions: CRQs

12 CRQs to be answered in 2 hours

Anatomy

1. Below is an image of the anterior chamber angle as viewed by gonioscopy.

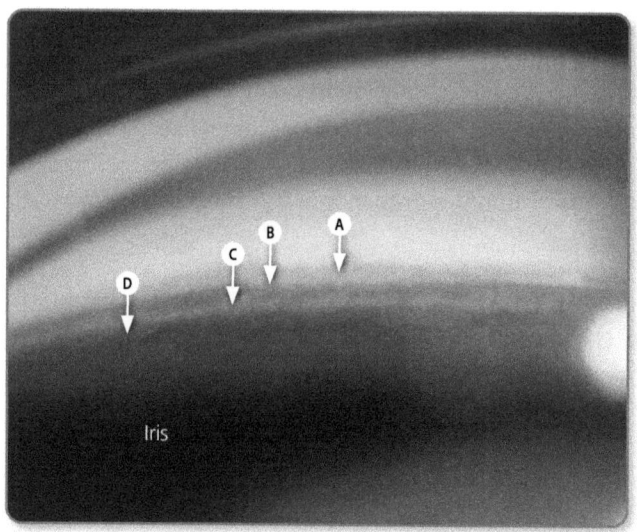

(a) Identify the structures labelled A–D. (4 marks)
(b) Describe the route of aqueous outflow via the conventional pathway. (3 marks)
(c) What effect does a rise in intraocular pressure have on the drainage via the non-conventional (uveoscleral) pathway? (1 mark)
(d) What is the mechanism by which pilocarpine reduces intraocular pressure in open angle glaucoma? (1 mark)
(e) Name a class of medications which increase outflow through the non-conventional pathway without directly altering aqueous production. (1 mark)

Pharmacology

2.

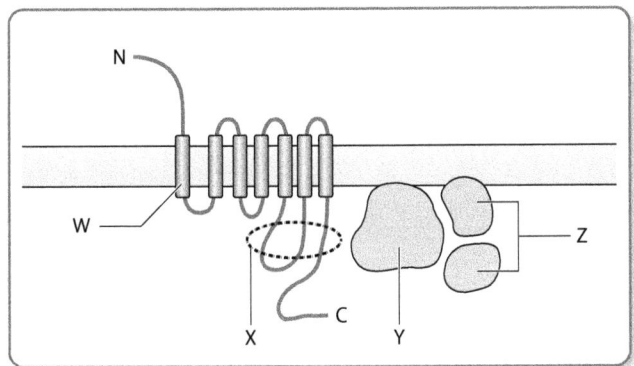

(a) What type of receptor is this? (1 mark)
(b) Name the structures labelled W to Z in the figure. (2 marks)
(c) Explain the importance of this type of receptor in rod photoreceptor cells, including how it is activated and the process triggered by its activation. (4 marks)
(d) Name three classes of intraocular pressure-lowering drugs which target this type of receptor. (3 marks)

Investigations and imaging

3.

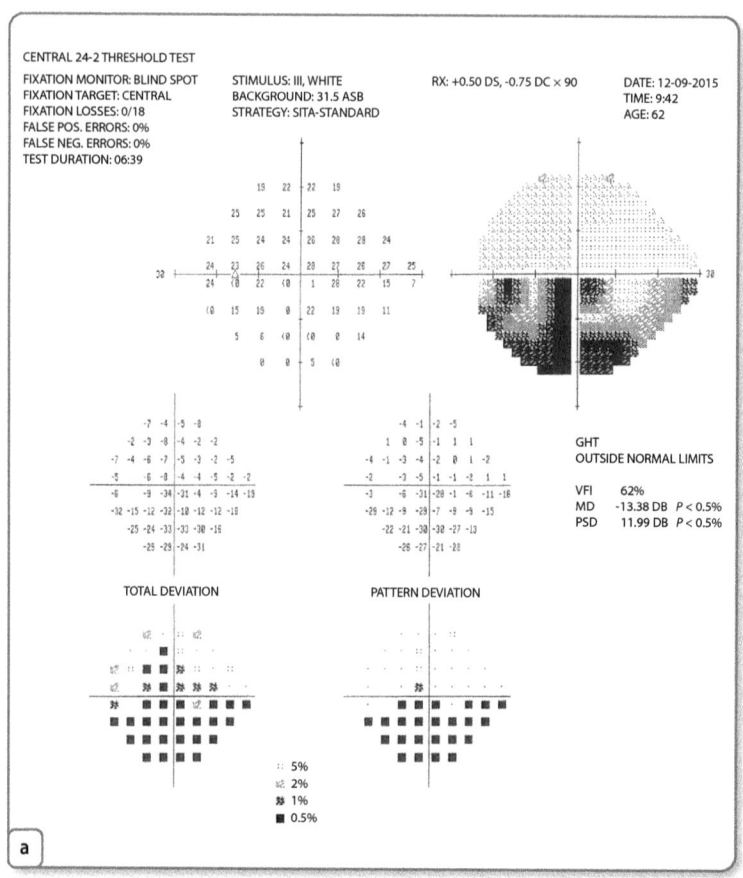

a

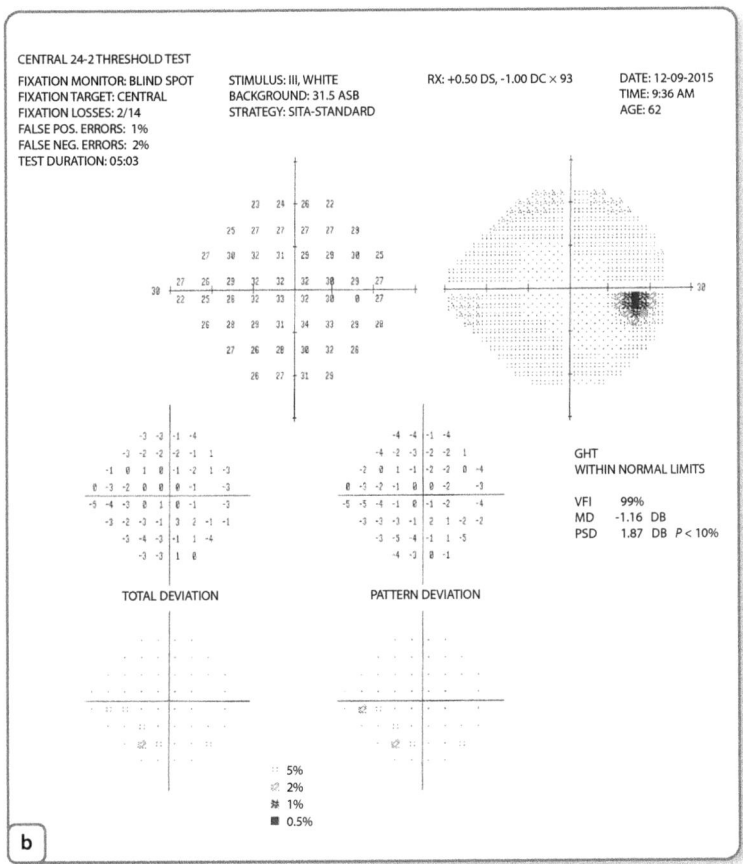

(a) The test comes from a Humphrey field analyser. What type of visual field test is this? (1 mark)
(b) Please comment on the reliability of this field test. (2 marks)
(c) What does pattern standard deviation (PSD) mean? (1 mark)
(d) Explain why the units of the numerical display of the visual field are decibels. (2 marks)
(e) Describe the field defect shown. (1 mark)
(f) Where in the visual pathway is the lesion most likely to be? (1 mark)
(g) Give a differential diagnosis for the field defect shown. (2 marks)

4. A 45-year-old woman attends the emergency eye clinic with a recent history of sudden, painless loss of vision in the left eye. Fundal examination shows signs of a central retinal vein occlusion.

She is normotensive with no known cardiovascular risk factors. Systemic enquiry reveals an episode of arthritis affecting the knees last year, as well as lethargy, mouth ulcers and a rash on sun-exposed areas triggered by bright sunlight. She explains that the general practitioner (GP) had found a raised erythrocyte sedimentation rate (ESR) when investigating her joint pains, but was simply monitoring it as her symptoms had improved.

Further blood tests are taken, the results of which are shown in **Table 2.1**.

Table 2.1 Screening blood test results*

Test	Result	Normal range	Units
Haemoglobin	121	115–165	g/L
White cell count	4.2	4.0–11.0	$\times 10^9$/L
Neutrophils	3.2	2.0–7.5	$\times 10^9$/L
Lymphocytes	**1.0**	1.5–4.5	$\times 10^9$/L
Platelets	**95**	150–400	$\times 10^9$/L
ESR	**38**	0–23 (varies with age and laboratory)	mm/h
CRP	<1	<8	mg/L
ANA	**Detected (1:640)**		
Cholesterol	4.0	3.9–6.0	mmol/L
Glucose (random)	5.5	3.5–11.0	mmol/L
Sodium	140	135–145	mmol/L
Potassium	4.6	3.5–5.0	mmol/L
Urea	6.0	3.5–6.5	mmol/L
Creatinine	115	60–125	mmol/L
IgG immunoglobulins	**18**	6–15	g/L
Protein electrophoresis	No paraproteins detected		

*Abnormal results in bold.
(ANA: antinuclear antibodies; CRP: C-reactive protein; ESR: erythrocyte sedimentation rate)

(a) What is the most likely diagnosis? (1 mark)
(b) What further blood test could you perform to support the diagnosis? (1 mark)
(c) Please give two other ophthalmic manifestations of this condition. (2 marks)
(d) Based on the results available, is the rise in IgG (immunoglobulin G) a monoclonal or polyclonal expansion? Why? (2 marks)
(e) Please state the mechanisms by which this condition can cause retinal vein occlusion. (2 marks)
(f) State two complications of central retinal vein occlusion. (2 marks)

5. A 45-year-old man presents with a 3-month history of headache and a 1-week history of increasing horizontal binocular diplopia. Papilloedema was seen on examination. An image from his MRI scan is shown below.

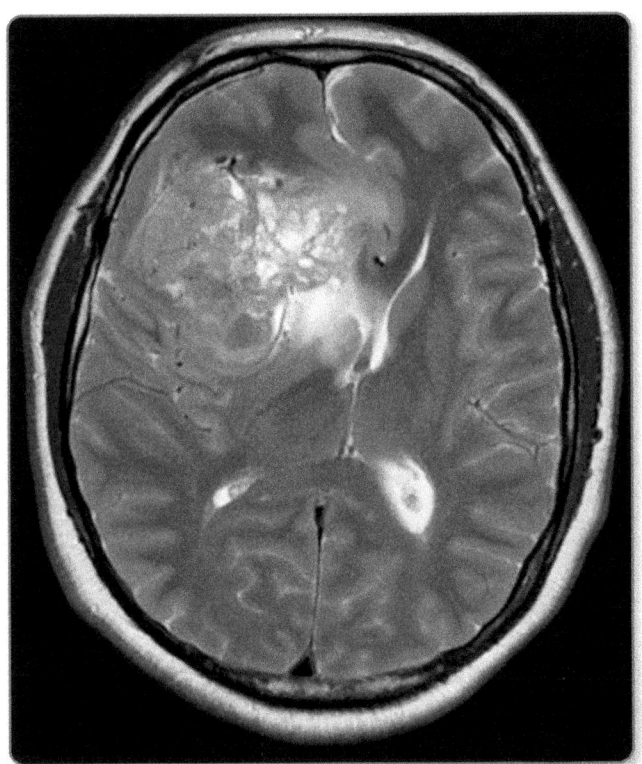

(a) Which particle is responsible for the signal measured in MRI? (1 mark)
(b) Which basic sequence is used in this MRI? (1 mark)
(c) State four advantages of MRI over CT for imaging the brain and cranial tissues. (4 marks)
(d) What three signs of mass effect can be seen in this image? (3 marks)
(e) The scan is reported as showing a probable vascularised meningioma over the right sphenoid wing with no involvement of the cavernous sinus or orbit. What is the most likely cause of his horizontal binocular diplopia? (1 mark)

6.

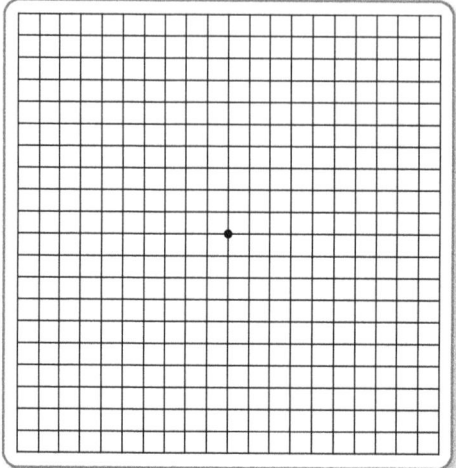

(a) What is the name of the test shown above? (1 mark)
(b) Describe how this test is performed. (5 marks)
(c) Below is a second chart. What is the purpose of the cross through the grid? (1 mark)

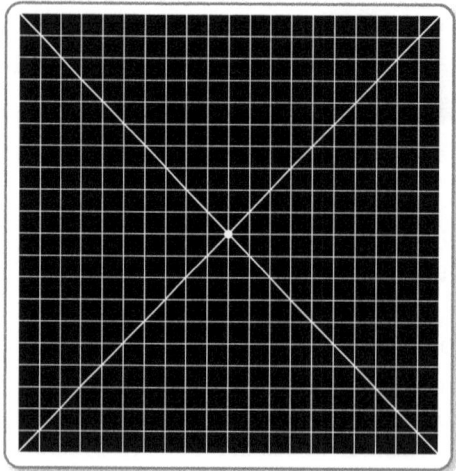

(d) How would you explain 'environmental' self-testing for distortion to a patient? (3 marks)

Microbiology

7. A patient at a UK hospital returns 24 hours after a routine left cataract extraction with a painful red left eye and severely reduced vision. They have no significant comorbidities. A vitreous biopsy is taken. Initial Gram stain and microscopy shows pink/red bacteria.

   (a) Describe the principles of the Gram stain technique. (5 marks)
   (b) Give the full names of two likely species given the results of the Gram stain and microscopy. (2 marks)
   (c) What is likely to be the principal type of inflammatory cell seen in the vitreous at this stage? (1 mark)
   (d) This patient has a severe allergy to penicillin. Which intravitreal antibiotic could be used that is likely to cover this organism? (1 mark)
   (e) Why is intravenous administration of this antibiotic unlikely to be effective? (1 mark)

Pathology

8.

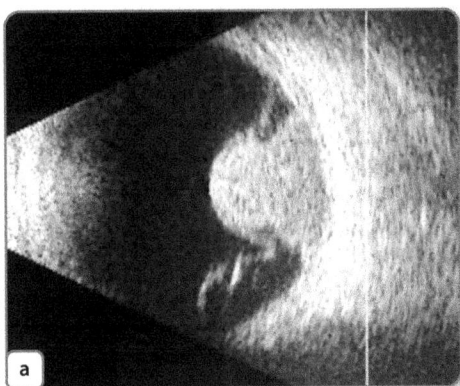
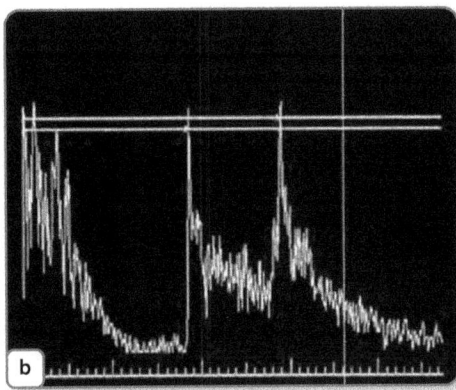

   (a) Which investigations are shown in Figures a and b above? (1 mark)
   (b) Please explain the principles behind these investigations. (3 marks)
   (c) Describe the abnormality shown. (2 marks)
   (d) What is the likely diagnosis? (1 mark)
   (e) Please give three pathological or cytogenetic factors associated with a poor prognosis. (3 marks)

Optics

9.
   (a) Draw a ray diagram of a focimeter with a test lens inserted and the instrument adjusted to neutralise it. (4 marks)
   (b) Why is the orientation of glasses in the focimeter important? (1 marks)
   (c) Two sets of line foci are seen in a focimeter as per the images below. What is the power of the lens? You may express your answer in plus or minus cylinder format. (3 marks)

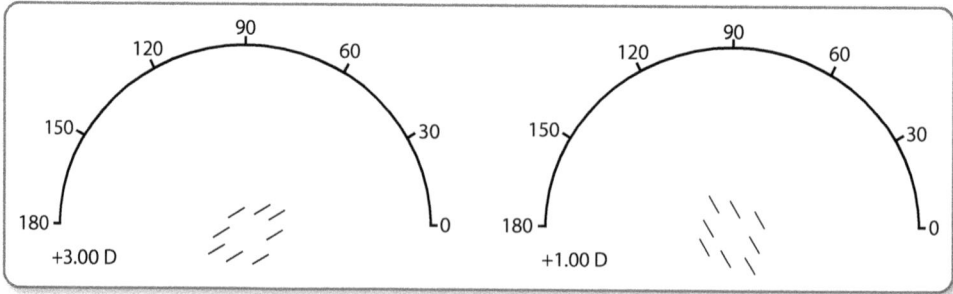

   (d) In lens neutralisation a lens is held above a cross on a piece of paper so that the cross is continuous through the lens (**Figure A**). When it is moved the cross moves with it (**Figure B**). Rotating the lens has no effect. What can be said about the sphere and cylinder prescription of this lens? (1 mark)

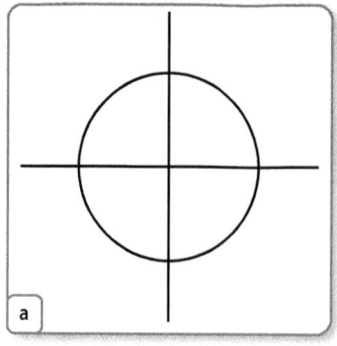
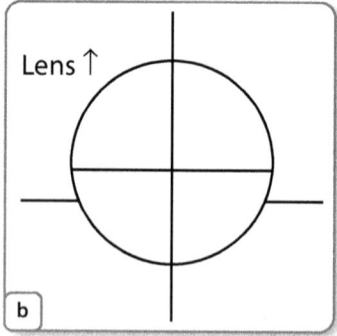

   (e) Another lens is held above the cross. Regardless of whether the lens is moved up or down the cross appears displaced downwards (**Figure c**). What can be said about this lens? (1 mark)

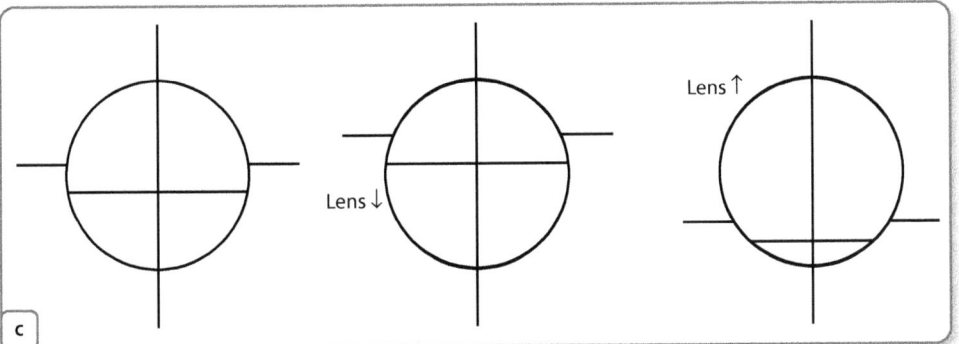

c

10. An 84-year-old man presents with a gradual, marked decline in his vision over 2 years. He particularly struggles with reading and recognising faces. His best corrected visual acuity (distance and near) is: 6/24, N36 right, 6/36, >N48 left.

Following a diagnosis of dry age-related dry macular degeneration (AMD), he is referred to the low vision clinic.

(a) What is the pathogenesis of dry AMD? (2 marks)
(b) Briefly outline the principles of action of magnifiers as low vision aids. (1 mark)
(c) Draw a ray diagram to show how a convex lens may be used to act as a simple magnifier. (3 marks)
(d) Galilean telescopes can be used as low vision aids. Please draw a ray diagram of a Galilean telescope. (4 marks)

11. Please answer the following questions regarding lasers.

(a) What does the acronym LASER stand for? (1 mark)
(b) Name three typical properties of a laser beam. (3 marks)
(c) With the aid of a diagram, illustrate how a laser beam is produced. (4 marks)
(d) Name two types of laser used therapeutically in ophthalmology (excluding corneal or refractive laser), stating the active medium and procedure(s) for which they are used. (2 marks)

Statistics and evidence-based medicine

12. The results of a hypothetical new test for glaucoma are given in **Table 2.2**. You may use a calculator for this question.

Table 2.2 Results of a new hypothetical test for glaucoma		
	Glaucoma patients	Patients without glaucoma
Test positive	950	100
Test negative	50	900
Total	1,000	1,000

(a) What is the false positive rate for this test? (1 mark)
(b) Calculate the sensitivity and specificity of this test. Showing your working. (2 marks)
(c) Calculate the positive and negative predictive values of this test. Showing your working. (2 marks)
(d) This test is being assessed as a screening tool for glaucoma in two different populations, both of 1 million people. Assume that in Birmingham, the prevalence of glaucoma is 1%, and in Marseille, the prevalence is 10%. In which population is a positive test result more useful for an individual patient? Please explain your answer. (3 marks)
(e) Name two ophthalmic conditions that are systematically screened for in the United Kingdom. (2 marks)

Answers: SBAs

Anatomy

1. **B It opens into the inferior meatus through the hiatus semilunaris**

    The maxillary sinus opens into the middle meatus of the nose (see Table 1.1, page 33) through small openings in the hiatus semilunaris. It is lined by mucoperiosteum, with the resulting mucus draining into the nasal cavity aided by the action of the epithelial cilia. Like the other paranasal sinuses, histologically the lining is pseudostratified columnar ciliated epithelium.

    The nerve supply is by the infraorbital nerve (a branch of the maxillary division of the trigeminal nerve), which travels through the roof of the sinus, and by the anterior, middle and posterior superior alveolar nerves. Hence, pathology of the maxillary sinus can result in pain felt in the teeth or cheek.

2. **A Blowout fractures of the orbit typically present with diplopia and exophthalmos**

    The ethmoid bone is paper thin, and thus trauma of little force can result in a medial orbital wall fracture. In orbital fractures, a communication between the sinuses and orbit is often created, such that nose blowing can force air into the periorbital tissues causing lid swelling.

    Blowout fractures refer to orbital fractures resulting from blunt trauma with an intact orbital rim. They typically present with diplopia and/or **enophthalmos**, which may initially be masked by periorbital swelling and bruising. Numbness of the cheek or infraorbital area suggests injury to the infraorbital nerve, which is a branch of the trigeminal nerve (maxillary division). The infraorbital groove, housing the infraorbital neurovascular bundle, runs in the maxilla near the thinnest and therefore most vulnerable part of the orbital floor.

3. **D All of the above**

    The inferior orbital fissure lies in the lateral orbital floor between the greater wing of the sphenoid and the maxilla. It is an opening into the orbital cavity from the infratemporal and pterygopalatine fossae, and should not be confused with the infraorbital foramen. The following structures pass through the inferior orbital fissure:

    - The inferior branch of the inferior ophthalmic vein, which passes out of the orbit and drains into the pterygoid venous plexus
    - The infraorbital artery and vein

- Two branches of V2, the maxillary division of the trigeminal nerve:
  i. The infraorbital nerve (the continuation of the maxillary nerve as it passes into the orbit)
  ii. The zygomatic nerve (which divides from the maxillary division immediately after it emerges from the foramen rotundum in the pterygopalatine fossa)
- Branches of the pterygopalatine ganglion

4. **B The eyebrows are drawn medially by contraction of the corrugator supercilii muscle, which is supplied by the fifth cranial nerve**

The principal muscles that are employed to move the eyebrows are the frontalis, which raises them; orbicularis oculi, which lowers them; and corrugator supercilii, which draws them medially towards the nose. All of these muscles, which form part of the muscles of facial expression, are supplied by the seventh cranial nerve. The other statements are true (the angular vein arises at the confluence of the supraorbital and supratrochlear veins).

5. **A Orbital cellulitis refers to post-septal infection**

The orbital septum forms a fibrous barrier, separating the anterior portion of the eyelids from the orbit. The septum is important clinically in cases of cellulitis, where a distinction is made between post-septal infection (orbital cellulitis) and pre-septal infection (often called periorbital cellulitis).

The lacrimal sac lies anterior to the orbital septum. For this reason, dacryocystitis typically causes pre-septal cellulitis and often settles with oral antibiotics (although surgery may be needed subsequently to prevent recurrence).

The tarsal plates (or tarsus) give firm structure to the lids, and measure around 10 mm in height in the upper lids, and 4–5 mm in the lower. The orbital septum attaches to the border of the tarsus.

There are approximately 100–150 eyelashes in the upper lid and 50–75 in the lower lid.

6. **D Orbital floor**

The inferior oblique muscle is the only extraocular muscle that does not arise at the orbital apex. It originates from the orbital plate of the maxilla, on the medial side of the orbital floor, posterior to the orbital margin. It arises lateral to the nasolacrimal groove, and in some cases is attached to the fascia covering the lacrimal sac. It passes inferior to the globe and inferior rectus, and inserts posterolaterally on the sclera, deep to the lateral rectus.

The superior oblique muscle originates just outside the common tendinous ring, from the periosteal covering of the sphenoid around the juncture of the body and the lesser wing. It passes through the trochlea, a cartilaginous pulley attached to the frontal bone, then under the superior rectus, and also inserts posterolaterally on the globe.

Therefore, unlike the recti, both oblique muscles insert posterior to the equator of the globe, on the temporal side.

7. A 1:2 to 1:7

A motor unit consists of a motor neuron and the muscle fibres that it innervates. Each motor neuron branches within the muscle to synapse on several muscle fibres. A motor unit contains a single type of muscle fibre.

The extraocular muscles have very small motor units compared to skeletal muscles elsewhere in the body, with an innervation ratio of approximately 1:2 to 1:7 – i.e. fewer than 10 muscle fibres in each motor unit. By contrast, the gastrocnemius muscle in the lower leg has an innervation ratio of approximately 1:1,000 to 1:2,000. An action potential generated by the neuron causes all the muscle fibres in the motor unit to contract together. Thus, smaller motor units allow for more precise movements.

8. A Craniopharyngioma: superior bitemporal field defect

Lesions of the optic chiasm typically cause a bitemporal hemianopia due to compression of the decussating fibres from the nasal retina, but the site of the lesion determines which fibres are affected first.

Visual fields that appear 'neurological', such as those in **Table 2.3**, can also have bilateral ocular causes. For example, binasal field defects, which are rare, may be caused by bilateral temporal retinal pathology.

Craniopharyngiomas can cause a range of field defects depending on their precise location, but are not commonly associated with superior bitemporal field defects.

Table 2.3 Visual field defects

Visual field defect	Site of lesion	Example
Superior bitemporal	Inferior to chiasm	Pituitary adenoma (may also cause a junctional scotoma)
Inferior bitemporal	Superior to chiasm	Suprasellar or olfactory groove meningioma
Junctional scotoma	Anterior to chiasm at the junction of the optic nerve	Sphenoid wing meningioma
Binasal	Lateral to chiasm	Hydrocephalus

9. B Around the conjunctival fornix

The accessory lacrimal glands of Krause are located around the conjunctival fornix. The similar accessory glands of Wolfring (also known as Ciaccio's glands) lie at the border of the tarsal plate at the opposite end to the lid margin.

10. C Posterior auricular artery

The posterior auricular artery is the 6th branch of the external carotid, arising after the occipital artery. There are many and varied mnemonics for the branches of the external carotid artery, one of which is Some Anatomists Like Freaking Out Poor Medical Students:

S – Superior thyroid artery

A – Ascending pharyngeal artery

L – Lingual artery

F – Facial artery

O – Occipital artery

P – Posterior auricular artery

M – Maxillary artery

S – Superficial temporal artery

Note that as the maxillary artery and superficial temporal artery are the terminal branches of the external carotid artery their order in the mnemonic can be reversed.

11. **D Left third nerve nucleus**

The oculomotor nucleus supplies the ipsilateral inferior rectus, inferior oblique and medial rectus. It also supplies the contralateral superior rectus from the superior rectus subnucleus. These motor fibres decussate within the third nerve nucleus and join the contralateral oculomotor nerve fascicle. The levator palpebrae muscles are supplied bilaterally by a central caudal subnucleus. Thus, a left third nerve nucleus lesion will affect the left inferior rectus, inferior oblique and medial rectus, the right superior rectus (sometimes both superior recti) and both levator palpebrae (though the ipsilateral side is usually more markedly ptotic).

12. **B Lateral rectus**

There are typically seven anterior ciliary arteries in each orbit, and these pass along the four rectus muscles providing a blood supply to each muscle before piercing the sclera to connect with the major arterial circle of the iris. The lateral rectus has only a single anterior ciliary artery, whereas the other rectus muscles have two each.

13. **C The inner third of the retina is supplied by branches of the central retinal artery whereas the outer two-thirds is supplied by the choroidal circulation**

Branches of the central retinal artery supply the inner two-thirds of the retina, whereas the outer third is supplied by the choroidal circulation. There is a watershed between the two circulations at the outer plexiform layer. The other statements above are true. In particular, it is worth noting that the choroidal circulation has a high rate of flow through a fenestrated capillary bed, providing nutrients and draining metabolites and waste, whereas the retinal circulation has a relatively low flow rate and a higher rate of oxygen exchange than the choroidal circulation.

14. B Anterior hyaloid face and posterior lens capsule

Wieger's ligament connects the anterior hyaloid face to the posterior lens capsule. It is circular or oval in cross-section, and 8–9 mm in diameter. Its adherence to the posterior capsule becomes weaker with age. Intracapsular cataract surgery in young patients almost invariably leads to vitreous loss because of the adherence of Wieger's ligament.

15. B 8–10 mm

The lacrimal canaliculi have a 2 mm vertical segment (the ampulla) followed by an 8–10 mm horizontal segment. The horizontal segments unite in over 90% of the population to form a common canaliculus before entering the lacrimal sac.

16. B The lamina fusca lies immediately superficial to the scleral stroma

The lamina fusca lies deep to the scleral stroma. It is a pigmented layer with a high density of melanocytes (its name is derived from the Latin *fuscus*, meaning 'dark'). These melanocytes may migrate through the emissary canals (which permit the passage of ciliary vessels and nerves) and clinically may give rise to pigmented spots on the episclera, typically 3–4 mm from the limbus (most commonly seen superiorly). The fascia bulbi covers the sclera and separates it from the orbital fat. It is often known as Tenon's capsule. The sclera is thinnest behind the insertions of the extraocular muscles (0.3–0.4 mm) and thickest posteriorly near the optic nerve (1 mm). At the limbus, it is approximately 0.8 mm thick.

17. A Ethmoid

The pterygopalatine fossa lies posterior and inferior to the orbit. The principal bony anatomical boundaries are listed in **Table 2.4**.

Table 2.4 Principal bony anatomical boundaries of the pterygopalatine fossa

Aspect	Boundary
Anterior	Posterior surface of maxilla
Posterior	Sphenoid including pterygoid process and greater wing
Superior	Sphenoid at the junction of the body and greater wing, orbital process of the palatine bone
Inferior	Pyramidal process of the palatine bone, open to palatine canals
Medial	Vertical (perpendicular) plate of the palatine bone
Lateral	Open to the infratemporal fossa via the pterygomaxillary fissure

18. A Aortic arch

The left common carotid artery generally arises directly from the aortic arch, whereas the right common carotid artery arises from the brachiocephalic trunk where it divides into the right common carotid and right subclavian arteries. There is a degree of anatomical variation, and in some individuals the left common carotid originates either with or from the brachiocephalic trunk (sometimes erroneously referred to as a "bovine arch"). However, these cases are the minority.

19. **D The transition between the neuroretina and the non-pigmented ciliary epithelium occurs at the ora serrata**

    There is an abrupt transition at the ora serrata from the inner non-pigmented ciliary epithelium to neuroretina. The epithelium of the ciliary body has an inner non-pigmented layer and an outer pigmented layer arranged apex to apex (a consequence of the embryology of the ciliary body epithelium, which is derived from an infolding of the optic vesicle). The inner non-pigmented ciliary epithelium is continuous anteriorly with the pigmented posterior epithelium of the iris, and its basement membrane is continuous posteriorly with the internal limiting membrane of the retina. The outer pigmented ciliary epithelium is continuous anteriorly with the anterior myoepithelium of the iris and posteriorly with the retinal pigment epithelium, and its basement membrane is continuous with Bruch's membrane.

20. **B Insertion of the recti**

    The most vulnerable sites to globe rupture are:

    - Where the sclera is thinnest: at or just posterior to the insertion of the rectus muscles
    - At the corneoscleral junction (limbus)
    - At the site of previous surgical incisions.

    Due to these vulnerable locations, the site of globe rupture is more commonly anterior to the equator.

    Globe ruptures occur more often in the left eye, as a significant proportion are due to assault by a right-handed assailant.

21. **A 250 µL**

    The normal fluid volume of the anterior chamber in most reference ranges is approximately 250 µL, although some studies have suggested a slightly lower in vivo volume. The anterior chamber is bordered anteriorly by the corneal endothelium and posteriorly by the iris and pupillary portion of the lens. The posterior chamber varies significantly with accommodation and has a fluid volume in the order of 60 µL.

22. **B Choriocapillaris**

    The choriocapillaris, the capillary layer of the choroid, consists of relatively wide-bore capillaries. Unlike the larger vessels in Haller's and Sattler's layers, the endothelium is fenestrated, rendering it permeable to large molecules including fluorescein. Fenestrations are transcytoplasmic holes in the endothelial cell (not gaps between the cells), typically 60–100 nm in size. Therefore, the diffuse leakage of fluorescein dye normally seen on fluorescein angiography occurs primarily from the choriocapillaris.

Biochemistry

23. A Erythrocyte

Mitochondria are organelles which are key to intracellular oxidative phosphorylation, in addition to several other metabolic functions. Sperm contain large numbers of mitochondria, but these are excluded from the ovum at fertilisation and hence only maternal mitochondria are inherited in the offspring. Mammalian erythrocytes contain neither nuclei nor mitochondria, both of which are ejected during erythropoiesis.

24. B Anaerobic glycolysis

Glucose derived from the aqueous provides the main energy source for the metabolic processes in the lens. Only lens epithelial cells possess mitochondria and so this is the only place in the lens where the citric acid (Krebs) cycle can occur. Anaerobic glycolysis accounts for approximately 80% of glucose consumption in the lens. The end products of this are lactic acid, which diffuses out into the aqueous, and adenosine triphosphate (ATP).

The remainder of glucose in the lens is metabolised via the pentose phosphate pathway and, particularly under conditions of excess glucose, the sorbitol pathway.

25. B MMP-2 is primarily involved in forming new extracellular matrix

Matrix metalloproteinases (MMPs) in the cornea, which degrade extracellular matrix, are involved in both the maintenance of normal framework (principally MMP-2) and remodelling following injury. The latter role is performed by several different MMPs: MMP-1 (a collagenase), MMP-2 (a gelatinase) and MMP-3 (a stromelysin), which are all produced primarily by the stroma, along with MMP-9 (a gelatinase) produced primarily by the epithelium. MMP-9 is involved in corneal epithelial remodelling. For further information about MMPs, see question 25 in Chapter 1, page 39.

26. D Tight junctions

The junctions at the apex of the retinal pigment epithelial cells are part of the blood–retinal barrier. As such the cells are joined by tight junctions, which act as a barrier to paracellular diffusion of molecules. **Table 2.5** provides a summary of key characteristics of the main intercellular junctions.

Table 2.5 Key characteristics of the main intercellular junctions

	Tight junctions	Adherens junctions	Gap junctions
Alternative names	Zonulae occludentes	Desmosomes	–
Subtypes	–	Spot desmosomes Belt desmosomes (zonulae adherentes)	–
Gap between cells	Nil detectable	~20 nm	~2 nm
Key features	Prevent paracellular diffusion of all molecules	Provide adhesion between cells	Allow passage of signalling molecules between the cytoplasm of different cells
Examples in tissue	Apex of retinal pigment epithelial cells; non-fenestrated endothelial cells in retinal blood vessels	Epithelium; muscle	Muscle; hippocampus

27. A The aqueous

Fibrillins are glycoproteins which form the structural scaffold of extensible microfibrils. They play a key role in providing strength and elasticity to ocular connective tissues. They are a crucial component of the lens zonules and are also found in the lens capsule, the vitreous, and the stroma of most ocular tissues. Mutations in the gene coding for fibrillin-1 can produce Marfan syndrome.

28. D It utilises radioisotopes to label test targets

Enzyme-linked immunosorbent assay (ELISA) is a plate-based assay which can be both qualitative and quantitative. It can be used to detect either an antigen or an antibody, and is used to test for a wide variety of diseases including HIV. It can detect and quantify peptides, proteins, antibodies and hormones. It is highly sensitive and specific, although it may not detect a mutated antigen. Unlike radioimmunoassay, ELISA does not require the use of radioisotopes. Instead the antibodies (or antigens) are labelled with an enzyme (such as horseradish peroxidase) which induces a colour change in a substrate when present.

29. B Chromophore regeneration occurs in the retinal pigment epithelium

The human visual cycle involves phototransduction and the subsequent regeneration of visual pigment. 11-*cis* retinal (a chromophore) is covalently bound to opsins via a lysine residue on one of the transmembrane domains. Upon photon absorption, it undergoes photoisomerisation from 11-*cis* retinal to all-*trans* retinal, triggering the phototransduction cascade. All-*trans* retinal is converted to all-*trans* retinol in the photoreceptor outer segment before being transported to the retinal pigment epithelial cells, where it is reconstituted into the 11-*cis* retinal isoform (an isoform of vitamin A derived from carotenoids).

Answers: SBAs

30. C Glutamate

Whilst there are many other retinal neurotransmitters and neuromodulatory peptides, glutamate is the neurotransmitter at the synapses between the photoreceptors and bipolar and horizontal cells. This synaptic transmission occurs in the outer plexiform layer following phototransduction.

31. D It is flexible

Actin is an important component of the cytoskeleton. It is a protein in the form of a microfilament, 7 nm in diameter, and can exist in monomeric and polymeric forms. Unlike microtubules, which are larger and rigid, actin is flexible.

As well as providing structural support, actin is involved in cell motility, cell division, cell–cell interactions, contractility and the interaction of transmembrane and cytoplasmic proteins.

The nature and distribution of the actin microfilaments are influenced by a host of specialised actin-binding proteins.

Embryology, growth and development

32. D Zygote; morula; blastocyst

The zygote is formed from the union of male and female gametes. The zygote undergoes a series of cleavage divisions to form a mass of cells known as the morula. A cavity forms within the morula, creating a fluid-filled sphere of cells known as a blastocyst.

33. D Temporalis

The second pharyngeal arch is the basis for the development of the muscles of facial expression (including platysma), along with stylohyoid, stapedius and the posterior belly of the digastric muscle. They are all innervated by the facial nerve. Temporalis is a muscle of mastication and thus is derived from the first pharyngeal arch. Please see Table 1.4 (page 41) for a summary of the muscular contributions of the pharyngeal arches.

34. C The epithelium of the cornea

The epithelium of the cornea is derived from surface ectoderm. Mesoderm gives rise to the endothelial linings of the blood vessels of the eye, including the tunica vasculosa lentis. It also gives rise to the endothelial lining of Schlemm's canal, and all of the extraocular muscles.

35. D The sphenoid sinus normally appears 2 months after birth

The sphenoid sinus normally develops 2–3 years after birth and reaches its adult size around the age of 14 years. The ethmoid and maxillary sinuses are usually present at birth, whilst the frontal sinuses, although occasionally present at birth, usually appear at around 2 years after birth. They continue to develop well into and even following puberty. The maxillary sinuses are the first sinuses to appear (usually at 3–4 months' gestation) and are also the largest paranasal sinuses.

36. **D 34 weeks**

    The hyaloid vasculature develops between the 3rd and 8th week along with the primary vitreous.

    By 18 weeks, the hyaloid vessels, the tunica vasculosa lentis and the primary vitreous have typically begun to atrophy. As they regress, Cloquet's canal is formed.

    Blood flow in the hyaloid artery stops at around 30 weeks, and by this point it has ceased to be visible on ultrasound. By 34–35 weeks it has lost its connection to the optic nerve and has essentially disappeared, though fragments can take longer to resorb entirely.

Genetics

37. **C Macular dystrophy**

    Macular dystrophy is an autosomal recessive disorder. Granular, lattice and Reis–Buckler dystrophies are all autosomal dominant, resulting from mutations in the transforming growth factor-β-induced gene on chromosome 5q31 (as are Avellino dystrophy and Thiel–Behnke dystrophy).

38. **B Interphase; prophase; metaphase; anaphase; telophase**

    The correct sequence is: interphase; prophase; metaphase; anaphase; telophase. There is some debate as to whether interphase is a true part of mitosis, as it is a 'resting phase' whilst the cell prepares metabolically for mitosis. In prophase, the chromosomes become visible to light microscopy as the chromatin condenses. The centrioles begin to migrate to opposite ends of the cell. In metaphase, the chromosomes align centrally within the nucleus, guided by spindle fibres. In anaphase, the paired chromosomes divide and move to opposite ends of the cell. In telophase, new nuclear membranes form, creating two daughter nuclei, and the chromosomes disperse within these new nuclei.

39. **B It is associated with nephroblastoma (Wilms' tumour) in 90% of patients**

    Aniridia is a bilateral, congenital eye malformation characterised by hypoplasia or total absence of the iris. Other ocular features include nystagmus, cataracts and foveal/optic nerve hypoplasia, with later complications including keratopathy and glaucoma. Aniridia is most commonly caused by *PAX6* variants (mutations) on chromosome 11.

Approximately two-third of aniridia cases are inherited in an autosomal dominant pattern with no systemic associations. The remaining one-third arise sporadically as *de novo* variants.

Nephroblastoma (Wilms' tumour) is associated with deletion of the *WT1* locus adjacent to *PAX6*. Genitourinary malformations and intellectual disability may also occur alongside aniridia with this deletion; this is referred to as WAGR syndrome [Wilms' tumour–Aniridia–Genital anomalies–Retardation (intellectual disability)]. In the vast majority of cases, WAGR syndrome arises from a spontaneous variant, and 45–60% of patients with WAGR syndrome will develop Wilms' tumour.

A rare syndromic cause of aniridia is Gillespie syndrome, which is a triad of non-progressive cerebellar ataxia, intellectual disability and partial aniridia. Hypotonia is also common. The causative gene has recently been identified as *ITPR1*, with several reported inheritance patterns. The iris in Gillespie syndrome is distinctive, with the sphincter muscle and other tissue central to the collarette missing. The overall appearance is of a congenitally dilated pupil.

See also feedback to Paper 1, CRQ 3 (pages 73–75).

40. **B It involves denaturing the DNA**

    Polymerase chain reaction (PCR) is a technique for cloning and amplifying DNA molecules.

    Part of the target DNA sequence must be known in order to create two primers: short oligonucleotides with a sequence complementary to the 3' end of each strand of the target DNA (which they will therefore bind to). The target DNA is heated in order to denature it and separate the strands, in a mixture containing the primers, heat-resistant DNA polymerase enzymes and an abundance of all four deoxynucleotide triphosphates (dATP, dCTP, dGTP, and dTTP).

    After heating, the mixture is cooled, and where the primer has bound to the target strand, DNA polymerase will synthesise a new strand. Synthesis occurs in the 5' to 3' direction. Each cycle doubles the number of DNA molecules, so theoretically, 30 cycles results in 2^{30} identical copies of the target DNA molecule.

41. **D Translocation usually results in loss of DNA**

    Chromosomes are numbered in decreasing order of size, and so chromosome 6 is bigger than chromosome 13.

    The Giemsa stain is used in cytogenetics to show alternating light and dark bands on chromosomes (G bands), which are numbered and help to describe the position of gene loci. Other important descriptors of chromosome structure are the p (short) and q (long) arms, which extend from the centromere.

    Translocations involve the transfer of a chromosome segment to another, non-homologous chromosome. The exchange is usually, but not always, reciprocal. DNA is not usually lost (i.e. the translocation is 'balanced'), and a translocation may be clinically undetectable. However, the break may occur within a gene and alter its protein product, or surrounding genes may come under the influence of different promoters. Additionally, the children of parents with a translocation are at an increased risk of 'unbalanced' translocations, with either too many or too few genes. Children with unbalanced translocations are at an increased risk of developmental problems.

Inversions involve two breaks in one chromosome, with 180° inversion of the segment. This can interfere with chromosome segregation at meiosis and result in unbalanced gametes. The breakpoints may also occur within a gene, and alter its function as described above.

42. D X-linked conditions

The Hardy–Weinberg equilibrium describes the constancy of gene frequencies in a population from one generation to the next. For a gene with two alleles, it is expressed as:

$$p^2 + 2pq + q^2 = 1$$

where p and q are the frequencies of the two alleles of a gene (i.e. $p + q = 1$).

It only applies in randomly-breeding populations, in the absence of mutation, genetic drift and natural selection.

Mating between first cousins is an example of non-random breeding and increases the chance of homozygosity for deleterious recessive alleles.

The Hardy–Weinberg equilibrium can apply regardless of whether a condition is X-linked or autosomal.

43. A Apoptosis

The tumour suppressor gene *p53* is one of the key regulators of cell growth. It is mutated in over half of adult tumours, although with variable penetrance in the tumour.

The p53 protein is activated in response to various types of damage to a cell, including damage to its DNA. The final result of p53 activation is either cell cycle arrest (to prevent mitosis) and DNA repair, or apoptosis. The latter is triggered if the damage is irreparable.

44. C Coloboma

Ocular associations of Down syndrome (trisomy 21) include keratoconus, myopia (and its associated risks including retinal detachment), cataract and Brushfield's spots on the iris.

Colobomata are a feature of trisomy 13 (Patau syndrome). Trisomy 13 is also associated with cyclopia, with other developmental malformations of the cornea and anterior chamber, and with persistent hyperplastic primary vitreous.

45. C Retinal angiomata

Von Hippel–Lindau syndrome (VHL) is an autosomal dominant cancer syndrome due to a mutation in the *VHL* gene on chromosome 3.

Retinal angiomata (also known as capillary haemangiomata or retinal haemangioblastomata) are the cardinal ocular feature. These are visible on dilated fundoscopy, progressing from a small dot to a vascular mass. These can be treated with laser or cryotherapy and can cause retinal detachment.

Cerebellar haemangioblastoma is also a cardinal feature of VHL but not an ocular one. Other non-ocular features include renal cell carcinomas and phaeochromocytomas.

46. **C Metacentric**

    Metacentric chromosomes have centromeres located centrally on the chromosome, giving rise to two arms of roughly equal length. Examples in the normal human karyotype include chromosomes 1 and 3. If the two arms of the chromosome are unequal the chromosome is termed submetacentric. Acrocentric chromosomes have their centromere near one terminal end, giving rise to a short arm that is difficult to observe. Examples in the normal human karyotype include chromosomes 13, 14, 15, 21 and 22. Holocentric chromosomes have a centromere running the length of the chromosome, and telocentric chromosomes have a centromere located at the terminal end. Neither holocentric nor telocentric chromosomes are found in the normal human karyotype.

Immunology

47. **B Regulatory mechanisms preventing inappropriate complement activation include factor B**

    Complement proteins form an important immunological effector mechanism. Whilst most complement is produced by the liver, extrahepatic synthesis occurs in mononuclear phagocytes as well as some epithelial cells. The complement system functions as an enzyme cascade, where inactive zymogens are sequentially converted to their active enzyme form.

    The classical cascade is triggered by antibody–antigen binding, and by acute phase proteins such as C-reactive protein (CRP). The alternative pathway is initiated by binding of C3b to the surface of an organism, foreign material or damaged tissue. This, in turn, allows the binding of factor B (a plasma protein), and subsequent activation of the cascade. The third complement pathway is the mannose-binding lectin pathway, where mannose-binding lectin (a serum protein) binds to certain sugars on the surfaces of pathogens, triggering a cascade similar to the classical pathway.

    There are several regulatory mechanisms preventing inappropriate complement activity, including factor H and factor I (but not factor B), C1 inhibitor and sialic acid.

48. **C Killing of cells by NK cells involves necrosis induced by granzymes**

    The complement cascade ultimately produces a membrane attack complex (MAC). The C5b-6-7-8 complex binds to C9, the latter polymerising to form tubes in the lipid bilayer. This creates a pore through which ions and water (but not proteins) pass, resulting in cell death by osmotic lysis.

By contrast, cell death caused by cytotoxic T cells (which belong to the CD8$^+$ subset) and NK cells involves both pore formation and apoptosis (but not necrosis). Activated cytotoxic T cells release lysosomes containing both perforins and granzymes. Perforin polymerises to create a channel in the membrane with some similarity to the MAC. Perforin release is accompanied by granzymes which induce apoptosis.

49. **D They present predominantly intracellular antigens that have been degraded in endosomes**

Antigen presenting cells (APCs) are the only cells that express high levels of major histocompatibility complex (MHC) class II molecules constitutively. However, stimulation by cytokines such as interferon-γ can induce certain endothelial and epithelial cells to express MHC class II molecules and thus act as 'non-professional' APCs.

The peptides presented on the cell surface bound to MHC class II molecules are principally from the extracellular environment, having been taken up by the cell and degraded in endosomes. They are recognised by CD4$^+$ T helper cells.

50. **A Germline mutations**

The number of different, specific antibodies we are able to generate is far greater than the number of genes in the human genome. Equally, the diversity of T cell receptors is almost infinite and achieved by the same principles. The main factors that contribute to the diversity of antibodies are as follows:

Prior to the antibody encountering the antigen:

1. Multiple germline gene segments encode different heavy and light chains
2. Both heavy and light chains contribute to the antigen-binding site
3. Somatic recombination of gene segments occurs prior to transcription
4. Junctional diversification: random loss and gain of nucleotides occurs at the joining of V, D and J gene segments

After exposure to the antigen:

5. Somatic mutation (or hypermutation) which increases the affinity of the antigen-antibody binding (affinity maturation)
6. Isotype switching: the antibody binding site remains unchanged, but the isotype of immunoglobulin changes under cytokine control (e.g. IgM to IgG)

Note that factors 1 to 5 above are genetic mechanisms that form the antigen-binding site, whereas 6 determines the biological properties of the antibody (for example, whether it is membrane-bound or soluble).

Investigations and imaging

51. B Flash VEP requires the patient to be conscious

Visual-evoked potential (VEP) records the electrical response of the visual cortex to a changing visual stimulus and thus is an objective test of the visual pathways. Electrodes are placed over the occipital cortex and mid-frontal area (reference electrode). It is essentially a limited electroencephalogram (EEG).

The visual stimulus may include flash, pattern-reversal (a black and white chessboard pattern that reverses) and pattern onset/offset (a pattern is alternated with a diffuse background).

Flash VEPs are possible in unconscious or anaesthetised patients, but a pattern VEP requires cooperation and fixation. Abnormal chiasmal crossing is the electrophysiological hallmark of albinism.

Microbiology

52. D Hepatitis B surface antibody (HBsAb) IgG

Hepatitis B surface antibody (HBsAb) IgG indicates full immunity to hepatitis B, derived either from previous infection or from vaccination. HBcAb IgM and IgG do not confer protection, and a positive test for either of these indicates probable previous or current infection with the virus (HBcAb is often used in the screening of blood donations as it is present during the convalescent period following infection). HBeAb IgG (and IgM) may be seen both in patients who have recovered from hepatitis B infection and in some chronically infected patients. Not all variants of hepatitis B produce envelope antigen and therefore not all patients develop envelope antibody.

53. A Adenovirus

Adenovirus is a double-stranded DNA virus. Influenza A, coxsackie and measles are all single-stranded RNA viruses [influenza A belongs to the family Orthomyxoviridae, coxsackie is a Picornavirus ('pico RNA virus' meaning small RNA virus), and measles belong to the family Paramyxoviridae]. All of these viruses can cause conjunctivitis.

54. A Coagulase

Coagulase indirectly promotes the conversion of fibrinogen to fibrin, which coats the surface of the bacterium and helps to isolate it from host defence mechanisms, including phagocytosis. Streptokinase, hyaluronidase and collagenase promote bacterial spread. Streptokinase activates fibrinolysin and dissolves fibrin clots; hyaluronidase breaks down the extracellular matrix constituent hyaluronate; collagenase dismantles collagen.

55. **D Owl's eye inclusion bodies are suggestive of herpes simplex virus**

    Owl's eye inclusion bodies are a specific histopathological sign of cytomegalovirus infection. Inclusion bodies can be detected on light microscopy in haematoxylin and eosin (H&E) stained preparations, and may be present in the cytoplasm (predominantly RNA viruses), the nucleus (generally DNA viruses) or both (as in cytomegalovirus). Cowdry type A inclusion bodies are nuclear and can be seen in herpes simplex, varicella zoster and sometimes cytomegalovirus infection.

56. **D Gentamicin**

    Gentamicin (an aminoglycoside) interferes with bacterial protein synthesis by irreversibly binding to the 30S subunit of the bacterial ribosome (the 30S subunit is also targeted by tetracyclines). Chloramphenicol, occasionally known internationally as chlornitromycin, clarithromycin (a macrolide) and clindamycin (a lincosamide) all target the 50S subunit of the bacterial ribosome, although they are structurally dissimilar.

57. **B Gram negative bacteria are protected by an outer membrane composed of glycosaminoglycans**

    Gram negative bacteria are surrounded by an outer membrane which lies outside their cell walls, but it is composed predominantly of lipopolysaccharides. It provides a degree of protection against some host defence mechanisms and antibiotics. Peptidoglycans are common to essentially all bacteria, and act as a key structural component of the cell wall. A number of antibiotics target bacterial cell wall synthesis, including β-lactams (penicillins, cephalosporins, carbepenems, and monobactams) and glycopeptides. Gram positive bacteria have much thicker peptidoglycan cell walls than Gram negative bacteria, and this allows them to retain the crystal violet dyes during Gram-staining.

58. **A They activate the alternative complement pathway**

    Being lipopolysaccharides, endotoxins are not highly antigenic, in contrast to exotoxins which are proteins. However, endotoxins do activate the alternative complement pathway and can provoke a significant inflammatory reaction. They are capable of causing systemic effects including fever and septic shock.

    Endotoxins are derived from the cell wall of Gram negative bacteria and are released when bacteria die. However, Gram negative sepsis is not invariably accompanied by endotoxaemia.

59. **A Contact lens wear**

    Contact lens wear is the most commonly implicated risk factor for microbial keratitis, particularly with extended wear and poor contact lens hygiene. Ocular surface disease, such as dry eyes, is the most important risk factor in non-contact lens wearers. Other factors include surgical or non-surgical trauma to the cornea, and systemic factors such as diabetes and immunosuppression.

60. **C Chlorination of water kills *Acanthamoeba* cysts**

    Acanthamoeba is a genus of motile, single-celled eukaryotic micro-organisms. The term 'amoebae' applies to a diverse group of eukaryotic micro-organisms – not all from one taxonomic group – which are motile, altering their shape and 'crawling' by extending pseudopods. *Acanthamoeba* are protists. They are also often described as protozoa (although the term is not used in modern taxonomy).

    Acanthamoeba are free-living and ubiquitous, being found in soil, water and even air. There are many species; *Acanthamoeba polyphaga* and *Acanthamoeba castellanii* are known to cause keratitis. *Acanthamoeba* exist in two forms:

    i. Active trophozoites, which produce destructive enzymes to penetrate the cornea; and
    ii. Metabolically inactive cysts, which are very hardy and survive unfavourable conditions including chlorination of water.

61. **A An IgE-mediated immune response will be mounted**

    Toxocara is a helminth and an IgE-mediated immune response will be mounted. Whilst canine and feline faeces are the typical route of transmission, this is in the form of ova and not cysts. *Toxocara canis* and *Toxocara cati* are very common gastrointestinal roundworm infections in dogs and cats, respectively.

    Toxocara is typically acquired in young childhood, e.g. from playing with kittens or puppies, and may present with acute systemic illness (fever, pneumonitis, fits, and myocarditis). Systemic illness, known as visceral larva migrans, is rarely fatal. Ocular toxocara infection is generally unilateral in the form of posterior uveitis.

Optics

62. **C Porro prism**

    Porro prisms deviate the image 180° but do not transpose it left to right. Dove prisms cause no deviation, but invert the image without transposing left to right. Wollaston prisms split an incident beam of light into two polarised emergent beams at a fixed angle without dispersion. Fresnel prisms are a series of parallel small prisms of equal refracting angle which cause an equivalent prismatic effect to a single large prism of the same angle. See the ray diagrams in **Figure 2.1** below.

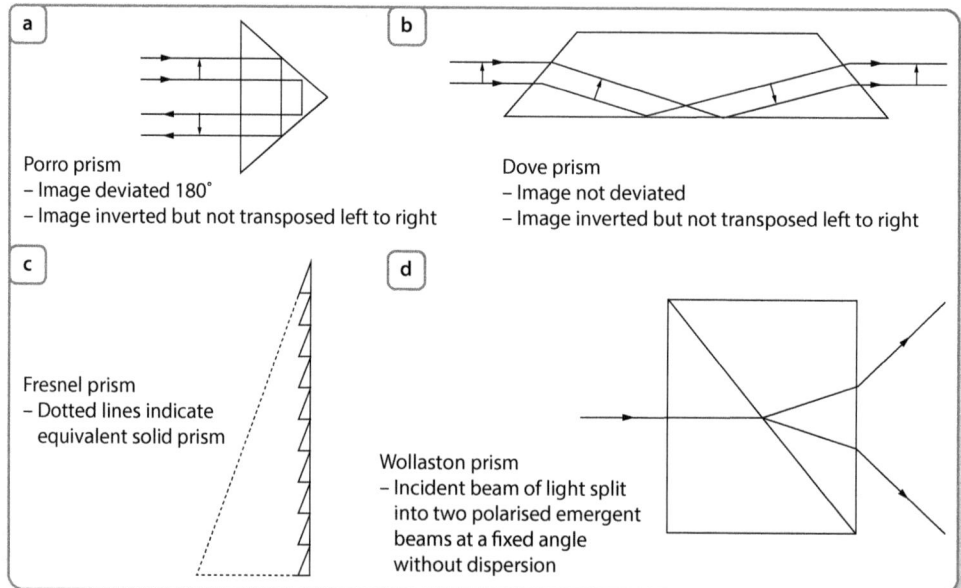

Figure 2.1 Ray diagrams for selected prisms.

63. **B** −3.75/−1.75 x 80° = −4.50/+1.75 x 170°

    To convert from positive to negative cylinder, or vice versa, simply add the given sphere and cylinder power together to give the new sphere, change the sign of the cylinder, and change the axis by 90°. It is important to be able to perform these calculations quickly and accurately.

64. **B Anterior chamber depth**

    The SRK formula was produced in 1980 by Sanders, Retzlaff and Kraff, and calculates the required power of intraocular lens for emmetropia with the equation:

    $$P = A - B(AL) - C(K)$$

    Where P is the required IOL power;

    A is a constant that is dependent on the model of lens used;
    B is a constant (calculated as 2.5);
    C is a constant (calculated as 0.9);
    AL is the measured axial length of the eye;
    K is the average keratometry.

    The SRK formula was found to be less accurate in eyes of atypical axial length, and a subsequent modification scale for the A constant was introduced depending on the axial length (the SRK II formula). A significant number of more complex formulae are now available in clinical practice, including the SRK/T and Hoffer Q, but these are not easily calculated by hand. See the answer to paper 1, CRQ 5 on page 76 for further discussion of lens formulae.

65. C 78 dioptres

Image magnification varies between different examination lenses and for this reason fundus measurements (for example, of optic disc size) should either be given with details of the lens used or corrected for the magnification factor. The magnification factors of some common lenses are given in **Table 2.6**.

Table 2.6 Magnification factors of some common fundus lenses	
Lens	Magnification factor
60 dioptre	1.15
66 dioptre	1.00
78 dioptre	0.93
90 dioptre	0.76

66. D 7.7

The radii of curvature of the anterior and posterior surfaces of the cornea are given as 7.7 and 6.8 mm respectively (Gullstrand measurements), although it is worth noting that in practice the radii of curvature vary both between individuals and depending on the location on the cornea. The three main refracting interfaces of the eye are the anterior cornea, and the anterior and posterior surfaces of the lens. The posterior corneal surface contributes much less than these three due to the fact that the corneal stroma and aqueous humour have similar refractive indices.

67. C 10

The loupe, or simple magnifying glass, is a convex lens. The relationship between magnification and dioptric lens power is governed by the following equation:

$$M = \frac{F}{4}$$

Where M is the magnifying power; F is the lens power in dioptres.

This can be rearranged to give the dioptric lens power, as follows:

$$F = 4M$$
$$= 4(2.5)$$
$$= 10 \text{ dioptres}$$

68. B Real, inverted, enlarged

When the object is between the centre of curvature (C) and the principal focus (F), the image formed by a concave mirror lies outside C, and is real, inverted and enlarged. Questions involving image formation by curved mirrors are straightforward if the basic rules for drawing the ray diagrams are followed (see **Figure 1.1** and answer to question 62, pages 49 and 50).

69. **C The first and second focal lengths of a contact lens are equal**

The vergence power (in dioptres) of a lens is the reciprocal of the second focal length (f_2) in metres. The shorter the focal length, the more powerful the lens. If the medium on either side of the lens is the same, then $f_1 = f_2$, but this is not the case with contact lenses which have air on one side and the tear film on the other.

70. **B 1.37**

The refractive index is a measure of the optical density of a medium. Light travels more slowly through a denser medium. The refractive index is based on the velocity of light through a particular medium compared to air. The absolute refractive index is the velocity of light in a medium compared to a vacuum. For example, air has a refractive index of 1, whereas diamond has a refractive index of 2.5, indicating that light travels 2.5 times slower through diamond than through air.

Some refractive indices are worth learning (**Table 2.7**).

Table 2.7 Refractive indices	
Medium	**Refractive index**
Air	1
Water/Aqueous/Vitreous	1.33
Cornea	1.37
Crystalline lens	1.38–1.41
Crown glass	1.52

71. **D Inversely proportional to the square**

Surface illumination is inversely proportional to the square of the distance from the light source. This is known as the inverse square law. In addition to this, it is of course directly proportional to the intensity of the light source.

The inverse square law also applies to other fields where a point source spreads its influence in all directions, such as gravity, sound and electric fields.

The reason the influence (in this case surface illumination) is inversely proportional to the square of the distance is because it spreads out in a sphere. As the distance from the light source increases, the area of the sphere of influence increases, and the influence at each point is diluted. The area of a sphere is $4\pi r^2$. The radius (r) is the distance from the light source, and so the surface illumination is inversely proportional to r^2.

72. **A A stereoacuity of 3,000 seconds of arc or better excludes significant amblyopia**

Stereopsis is depth perception derived from fusion of the slightly different images obtained from each eye. Panum's fusional area is an ellipse of space in which objects will appear as a single image, with the light stimulating both retinas simultaneously. The disparity in the position of the retinal images allows true stereopsis.

Stereoacuity of 60 seconds of arc or better is considered normal. Stereoacuity of 3,000 seconds of arc indicates the presence of gross stereopsis, but does not exclude significant amblyopia.

The Titmus stereoacuity test, which includes a large image of a fly (hence it is sometimes called the Wirt fly test), involves vectographs: the two superimposed views of the image are polarised at right angles to each other and the subject wears polarising glasses to see the composite image.

The TNO test requires red–green filter glasses. Frisby and Lang tests do not require special glasses.

73. **C 43**

    The overall refractive power of the average human eye is approximately 58 dioptres (D), the two refracting elements being the cornea and the lens. Based on Gullstrand's measurements, the dioptric power of the aphakic eye is 43 D. Note that in isolation the lens is calculated to have a power of 19 D, but the overall effect of removing the natural lens in vivo is actually only a 15 D reduction in the power of the eye (58–43 D).

74. **A An infrared filter in the eyepiece of the Nd:YAG laser allows the laser output to be seen as a red dot to facilitate aiming**

    The infrared filter in the eyepiece of the neodymium-doped yttrium aluminum garnet (Nd:YAG) laser is to protect the eyes of the operator. The red aiming beam is produced by a coaxial He–Ne laser.

    Argon blue light is absorbed by xanthophyll in the inner and outer plexiform layers of the macula, and therefore should not be used to treat lesions in this area.

    The distance between the reflectors in a laser tube is a multiple of the wavelength of the laser to allow for accumulation of photons that are in phase and parallel.

    The Nd:YAG laser has a wavelength of 1,064 nm, and therefore lies in the infrared spectrum.

75. **B 2.5 dioptres**

    The accommodative power required to focus on a particular point can be calculated by the formula:

    $$A = V - R$$

    Where A is the accommodative power required to focus on a point; V is the dioptric equivalent of the distance to the object (i.e. the reciprocal of the distance in metres); R is the dioptric equivalent of the far point distance (note this is positive for myopes, negative for hypermetropes, where it lies behind the eye, and zero for emmetropes).

$$A = V - R$$
$$A = \frac{1}{0.25} - 1.5$$
$$A = 4 - 1.5 = 2.5$$

Therefore, 2.5 dioptres of accommodation are required in this case.

76. D Image IV

Image IV is an inverted real image, as it is the reflection from a concave reflecting surface (the lens–vitreous interface). Images I, II and III are erect virtual images as they arise from convex reflecting surfaces (the air-cornea interface, cornea-aqueous interface and aqueous-lens interface respectively).

77. D Vitreous at the posterior lens surface acting as a doublet lens

The vitreous at the posterior lens surface does not act as a doublet lens. The anterior corneal curvature is steeper centrally than peripherally, and the lens nucleus has a higher refractive index than the cortex. Both of these features reduce spherical aberration. The position of the iris in front of the lens acts as a stop for incident light at the periphery of the lens, and therefore reduces spherical aberration at the retina. Another adaptation of the eye to reduce the effect of spherical aberration is the so-called Stiles–Crawford effect, where cone photoreceptors are more sensitive to axial/paraxial light than to oblique light from the peripheral cornea.

78. B It is used with its concave surface towards the observer

The Hruby lens is a planoconcave lens and is used with the concave surface towards the patient. It has a power of −58.6 dioptres. It forms a virtual, erect and diminished retinal image that lies within the eye of the patient but within the focal range of the slit lamp (usually in the pupillary plane when the lens is positioned close to the patient's eye). The lens and image position are illustrated in **Figure 2.2**.

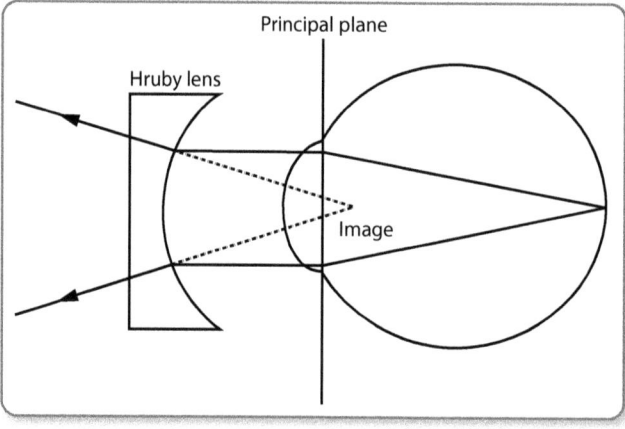

Figure 2.2 Hruby lens.

79. C +3.00 DS/+2.25 DC axis 85°

'With the rule' astigmatism is a term used when the steepest meridian of the eye is vertical. In order to correct this with glasses, the positive cylinder will be at or near 90° (or negative cylinder at 180°).

'Against the rule' astigmatism is therefore when the horizontal meridian of the eye is the steepest, i.e. the axis of the positive cylinder in the correcting lens is at or near 180°.

If the axis lies obliquely, such as in option (b), then this is neither 'with' nor 'against' the rule. This refers to axes between 30° and 60°, or 120° and 150°.

All of the above (with the rule, against the rule, and oblique astigmatism) are types of regular astigmatism, i.e. where the axes of the two meridians are at right angles to each other.

80. C 5 minutes of arc

The visual angle subtended by a letter on a Snellen chart at its specified distance is 5 minutes of arc (5'). The discernible components of a letter that allow it to be differentiated from other letters each subtend 1 minute of arc (1') and therefore, to recognise a letter, the eye must have a resolution of at least 1 minute of arc (**Figure 2.3**).

For those unfamiliar with these small angular measurements: there are 60 seconds of arc (") in a minute, and 60 minutes of arc (') in a degree (°).

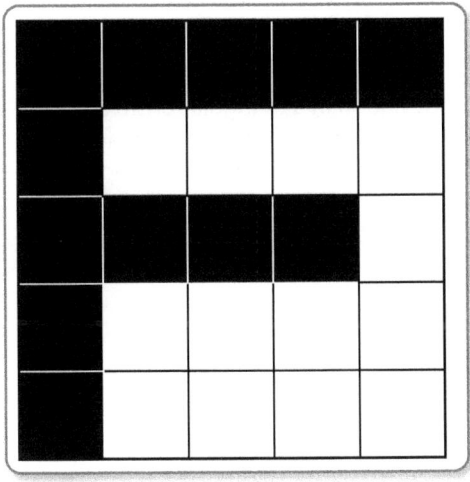

Figure 2.3 Snellen letter, each box representing 1 minute of arc.

81. C 10 cm

It is possible to calculate the dioptric power of a simple magnifying glass using the formula:

$$F = 4M$$

Where F is the power of the lens in dioptres and M is the magnification of the lens (note this is a modification of the same equation for calculating the magnifying power of a simple loupe, and assumes a near point of 25 cm).

Therefore, this magnifying glass has a power of:

$$4 \times 2.5 = 10 \text{ dioptres}$$

The lens to object working distance is the focal length of the lens which is the reciprocal of the dioptric power of the lens:

$$\frac{1}{10} = 0.1 \text{ m} = 10 \text{ cm}$$

At this distance the rays emerging from the lens are parallel and therefore, provided the patient is wearing the appropriate distance prescription, the size of the image will not vary with head movement.

82. A At the first principal focus

A convex lens produces an erect, virtual image at infinity when the object is located at the first principal focus. Remember that the second principal focus is behind the lens in a convex lens. It is always worth drawing the ray diagram for these questions. One ray runs from the top of the object parallel to the principal axis, and is refracted through the second principal focus (note in the case of concave lenses it is a virtual ray that passes through the second principal focus). The other runs from the top of the object through the principal point at the centre of the lens, and continues undeviated. The image is formed where these two rays intersect. See the diagrams on page 51, particularly Figure 1.2c.

83. D Width of prism base

The three factors controlling the angle of deviation in a triangular prism are: the angle of incidence of the light ray, the refracting angle of the prism and the refractive index of the prism material. Because refractive index varies depending on the wavelength of light, the angle of deviation is also indirectly dependent on the wavelength (and therefore frequency) of the incident light – hence the greater deviation of blue light than red light.

Pathology

84. D Retinoblastoma

Flexner–Wintersteiner rosettes are tumour cells arranged around a central lumen. The cells resemble primitive photoreceptor cells on electron microscopy. They are characteristically seen in retinoblastoma, as are Homer–Wright rosettes (which represent neuroblastic differentiation and are relatively non-specific) and fleurettes (which represent photoreceptor differentiation). Although characteristic of retinoblastoma, Flexner–Wintersteiner rosettes are not pathognomonic as they can also be seen in pineoblastomas and medulloepitheliomas.

Answers: SBAs

85. B Phacolytic glaucoma

The crystalline lens can induce glaucoma in several ways (**Table 2.8**).

Table 2.8 Types of lens-induced glaucoma	
Name	Mechanism
Phacoanaphylactic glaucoma	Delayed-onset granulomatous reaction induced by exposed lens fragments following trauma or surgery, with secondary glaucoma due to trabeculitis and/or blockage of trabecular meshwork by inflammatory cells
Phacolytic glaucoma	Obstruction of trabecular meshwork by engorged macrophages following leakage of lens protein through the lens capsule into the anterior chamber (typically in mature/hypermature cataracts)
Phacomorphic glaucoma	Enlargement of the cataractous lens causing pupillary block and secondary angle closure
Lens particle glaucoma	Acute obstruction of the trabecular meshwork by fragments of lens material

86. D Progression is generally most rapid in the fifth decade of life

Keratoconus is a non-inflammatory corneal degeneration which typically presents during adolescence and generally stabilises by the early to mid-thirties. It may be associated with systemic disease, including atopy, Down syndrome and Marfan syndrome. Eye rubbing increases the probability of disease progression.

Fleischer rings are the result of iron deposition in the basal epithelial layers at the base of the cone (not to be confused with Kayser–Fleischer rings which are due to copper deposition in Descemet's membrane caused by Wilson's disease and certain other hepatobiliary pathologies).

87. A Behçet's disease

Behçet's disease is characterised by infiltration with lymphocytes and plasma cells and does not cause a granulomatous reaction. Granulomatous inflammatory reactions are precipitated in response to several groups of stimuli: endogenous materials (e.g. chalazion); exogenous materials (e.g. suture granuloma); vasculitis [e.g. granulomatosis with polyangiitis (GPA) – formerly known as Wegener's granulomatosis]; sarcoidosis; autoimmune conditions (e.g. Crohn's disease); and a range of infectious stimuli (e.g. Lyme disease, syphilis, mycobacteria).

88. B Fibrosarcoma

Malignant tumours originating from mesenchymal cells have the suffix *-sarcoma*, whereas benign mesenchymal tumours have the suffix *-oma* (compare liposarcoma: malignant with lipoma: benign). Similarly, malignant tumours originating from the epithelial cells of surface tissues are denoted carcinomas (e.g. squamous cell carcinoma) and benign tumours are denoted papillomas (e.g. basal cell papilloma). Glandular epithelial cell tumours are called adenocarcinoma if malignant and adenoma if benign. Tumours derived from neuroectodermal cells are generally malignant, with a few notable exceptions including neurofibromas, ganglioneuromas and some meningiomas.

89. B Nerve fibre layer

Cotton wool spots occur in the retinal nerve fibre layer and are usually a sign of retinal ischaemia. Whilst non-specific, they are most commonly seen in diabetic retinopathy and retinal vein occlusions. Obstruction of axoplasmic flow in unmyelinated ganglion cell axons results in an accumulation of debris within the nerve fibre layer. This is seen as a small, fluffy white retinal lesion. Histologically, globular structures called cytoid bodies are seen on light microscopy. On fluorescein angiography they cause hypofluorescence.

90. D Spindle cell type

Choroidal melanomas are usually composed histologically of spindle cells (better prognosis), epithelioid cells (poorer prognosis) or (more commonly) a mixture of the two. Cytogenetic analysis of the tumour itself or a metastasis can give powerful prognostic information. The most important cytogenetic predictors of mortality and metastasis in choroidal melanoma are monosomy of chromosome 3 and duplication of 8q.

Older age, large tumour size and extrascleral extension are further poor prognostic factors.

91. C Subretinal lipid exudation

Following separation of the neurosensory retina from the retinal pigment epithelium, several pathophysiological changes occur, including:

- Degeneration of photoreceptors
- Proliferation and migration of the retinal pigment epithelium
- Subretinal recruitment of macrophages

Subretinal lipid exudation is not a typical feature of retinal detachment but does occur in wet age-related macular degeneration.

92. B Loose sutures

Corneal graft rejection is a type IV hypersensitivity reaction. Risk factors include:

- Young age
- Repeat grafts
- Large grafts
- Preoperative stromal vascularisation
- Loose or broken sutures
- Active inflammation

93. B Large hyphaema

Raised intraocular pressure (IOP) is common following blunt trauma due to many different mechanisms. There can be early and/or late rises in pressure following the injury.

Hyphaema is a common cause of early raised pressure due to obstruction of the trabecular meshwork (TM) by red blood cells and fibrin. Anterior chamber inflammation is very common, and the topical steroid given to treat this can also cause a (usually slower) rise in IOP.

Angle recession (indicating damage to the TM), peripheral anterior synechiae formation (causing angle closure) and vitreous haemorrhage (a risk factor for ghost cell glaucoma) are all causes of a late rise in IOP.

Pharmacology

94. **B The nicotinic acetylcholine receptor is an example of this type of receptor**

    The nicotinic acetylcholine receptor is a ligand-gated ion channel.

    G-protein-coupled receptors (GPCRs) are a large family of receptors whose members include the muscarinic acetylcholine receptor, adrenoreceptors and opioid receptors. GPCRs are a class of metabotropic receptors. They have a characteristic structure involving seven transmembrane domains and an intracellular coupling site for G proteins. G proteins have three subunits and are named after their affinity for guanine nucleotides. G proteins provide a link between the receptor and its intracellular effector systems, which include second messenger systems (such as adenylate cyclase/cAMP) and ion channels. The α subunit catalyses the hydrolysis of GTP to GDP, which terminates the signal.

95. **B In the presence of a competitive antagonist, the agonist logarithmic dose-response curve is shifted to the right**

    Drug antagonism can occur by different mechanisms, including pharmacokinetic antagonism, where one drug affects the body's handling of another, and physiological antagonism, where two drugs have opposite effects. However, receptor antagonism is where a ligand or drug binds to the same receptor as the agonist and blocks activation.

    Receptor antagonism can be broadly divided into competitive and non-competitive antagonism, and both of these can be reversible or irreversible. In competitive antagonism, the antagonist binds to the same site on the receptor as the agonist, therefore directly 'competing' with it. In non-competitive antagonism, the antagonist binds to a different site on the receptor to inactivate it. Reversible antagonists bind in a non-covalent manner, and will therefore dissociate from the receptor and can be 'washed out'. Irreversible antagonists bind covalently to the receptor, and will remain bound until the receptor is destroyed and replaced. Irreversible antagonists therefore cannot be 'washed out' or displaced.

    In the presence of a competitive antagonist, the agonist logarithmic dose-response curve is shifted to the right, i.e. higher doses of agonist are required to achieve the same response, but neither the gradient of the curve nor the maximum response is affected.

    Brimonidine is an example of a selective agonist at the $α_2$ adrenoceptor.

96. C Tamsulosin

Intraoperative floppy iris syndrome (IFIS) is characterised by a small pupil and billowing of the iris during cataract surgery, sometimes with iris prolapse through the corneal incision. It increases the risk of complications such as iris trauma and posterior capsular rupture.

The risk of IFIS is increased by certain α_1-antagonists, with the most common culprit being tamsulosin, which is widely prescribed for benign prostatic hypertrophy. As well as causing relaxation of the smooth muscle at the bladder neck, it also has long-term effects on the iris dilator muscle. Other α_1-antagonists, such as doxazosin and alfuzosin, also increase the risk of IFIS, but to a lesser extent.

The other agents listed in the question stem can precipitate acute angle closure but do not cause IFIS.

97. C The principal barrier to intraocular penetration is the corneal endothelium

The most common route of drug delivery to the eye is topical administration. Whilst a drop of topical medication is 50–100 µL, the conjunctival sac can only hold 15–30 µL, of which approximately 7 µL is already occupied by the natural tear film.

The main barrier to intraocular penetration of topical drugs is the corneal epithelium. Tight junctions between the superficial cells form a hydrophobic barrier, through which lipid-soluble drugs can pass. By contrast, the corneal stroma is hydrophilic, and only provides a barrier to highly lipophilic compounds. The endothelium is not a significant barrier to drug penetration, and is kinetically homogenous with the aqueous.

Excess lacrimation decreases trans-corneal drug absorption by dilution and loss of the drug. For this reason, topical ophthalmic medications are typically formulated at a physiological pH, despite the increased permeability of the cornea at high or low pH.

98. D Pyridostigmine

Atropine, cyclopentolate and ipratropium are all muscarinic antagonists whose potential systemic side effects include dry mouth, tachycardia, palpitations, and urinary retention. The first two agents are common topical mydriatics and cycloplegics, whereas ipratropium is used as an inhaled bronchodilator.

Pyridostigmine is an inhibitor of acetylcholinesterase, used in the treatment of myasthenia gravis. It enhances rather than blocks acetylcholine activity at parasympathetic synapses.

99. C Increased osteoblast function

Glucocorticoid corticosteroids have various metabolic effects, including:

- Hyperglycaemia, resulting from reduced uptake and utilisation of glucose along with an increase in gluconeogenesis; and
- Protein catabolism, and decreased protein synthesis, especially in muscle

Glucocorticoids increase the risk of osteoporosis by reducing bone formation by osteoblasts. Their influence on osteoclasts is more complex, as they have both direct and indirect effects on osteoclast differentiation and function, and differing effects in early and late stages of therapy.

Corticosteroids decrease fibroblast function, meaning that they can be beneficial in reducing the chronic inflammatory response, but that they also impair wound healing.

100. A Acetylcholinesterase inhibition

The Tensilon test (Tensilon is a brand name for edrophonium) is used to differentiate myasthenia gravis from other forms of neuromuscular weakness. Edrophonium inhibits acetylcholinesterase, therefore reducing the breakdown of acetylcholine in the synaptic cleft. This potentiates transmission at the neuromuscular junction and temporarily improves the muscle weakness in myasthenia patients (who have a reduced number and activity of nicotinic acetylcholine receptors at the neuromuscular junction due to autoantibodies to the receptor). The test has a sensitivity of approximately 60–80%.

Conversely, edrophonium will not significantly improve the muscle weakness in patients with Lambert–Eaton myasthenic syndrome, as the antibodies in this condition are directed against the presynaptic voltage-gated calcium channels and so the nerves fail to exocytose significant amounts of acetylcholine.

101. A DNA crosslinking

Mitomycin-C and 5-fluorouracil (5-FU) are antimetabolites which can both be used as an antiproliferative agent during glaucoma surgery to reduce scarring. They inhibit fibroblast proliferation via effects on DNA and RNA.

Mitomycin C is an alkylating agent which crosslinks DNA, inhibiting further DNA and RNA synthesis. 5-FU is a fluorinated pyrimidine analogue, which inhibits DNA and RNA synthesis and function without crosslinking. Mitomycin C provides a longer suppression of fibroblast proliferation than 5-FU, and is independent of the cell cycle phase of the fibroblasts at the time of application, whereas 5-FU is only effective at certain points in the cell cycle. Clinical studies have shown a lack of significant epithelial toxicity with mitomycin C when applied for a short duration, as in glaucoma surgery. Conversely, 5-FU causes significant toxic effects to the corneal epithelium.

102. B Low molecular weight heparins do not require routine monitoring, but can be monitored using anti-Xa levels if required

Intravenous unfractionated heparin (UFH) requires monitoring with the activated partial thromboplastin time (APTT). UFH can also be given subcutaneously and does not generally require monitoring in this situation other than in pregnancy. Low molecular weight heparins (LMWH) have a longer half-life: they are given subcutaneously and do not require routine monitoring. However, if monitoring of LMWH is needed, for example in renal failure (it is renally excreted) or pregnancy, anti-Xa levels are measured.

The international normalised ratio (INR) is the ratio of a sample's prothrombin time to a standard. The dose of warfarin is adjusted according to the results of the INR. Warfarin is teratogenic during the first trimester and should be avoided entirely throughout pregnancy.

In the last decade, the use of direct oral anticoagulant drugs (DOACs), including dabigatran, rivaroxaban, apixaban and edoxaban, has increased significantly. These medications act directly on proteins within the clotting cascade, in contrast to warfarin which acts as a vitamin K antagonist (therefore indirectly disrupting the clotting cascade). DOACs reach their peak effect much more rapidly (hours, as opposed to days for warfarin), have a lower rate of life-threatening intracranial haemorrhage, have fewer drug interactions, and do not require routine monitoring. However, reversal of their effects in the context of uncontrolled bleeding has proved challenging, although novel reversal agents have recently become available for some DOACs (including dabigatran, apixaban and rivaroxaban), and other agents are in development.

103. C Heroin

Heroin, as an opiate, will cause miosis rather than mydriasis. This is most likely via reducing cortical or brainstem inhibition of the Edinger–Westphal nucleus. Mydriasis can be brought about by either anticholinergic effects (inhibiting miosis) or adrenergic stimulation (potentiating mydriasis). Some common examples and their principal mechanisms are listed in **Table 2.9**.

Table 2.9 Mechanisms of mydriasis for common recreational drugs	
Drug	**Mechanism**
Amphetamine	Increased noradrenaline release
Cocaine	Decreased noradrenaline reuptake
MDMA	Increased release of monoamine neurotransmitters (including noradrenaline), inhibition of serotonin reuptake
(MDMA: 3,4-methylenedioxymethamphetamine)	

Physiology

104. C 500

The maximal spectral sensitivity of a photoreceptor is determined by its visual pigment (**Table 2.10**). S, M and L refer to short, medium and long wavelength sensitivity of the cones.

The maximal spectral sensitivity of rods (~ 500 nm) corresponds very closely to that of the dark-adapted retina. The maximal spectral sensitivity of the light-adapted retina is approximately 555 nm.

Table 2.10 Spectral sensitivity of photoreceptors	
Photoreceptor type	Wavelength of approximate peak spectral sensitivity (nm)
Blue (S) cones	445
Rods	500
Green (M) cones	545
Red (L) cones	570

105. B Dichromatism results in a reduced range of colour detection

The commonest congenital colour vision defect is deuteranomaly, which occurs in 5% of men and 0.3% of women. This is a form of anomalous trichromatism in which affected individuals have a relative deficiency in one of the three cone populations, resulting in a shift in the spectral sensitivity.

The other forms of anomalous trichromatism are tritanomaly and protanomaly.

By contrast, absence of a functioning cone population results in dichromatism, called tritanopia, deuteranopia or protanopia. Such individuals match all colours from a mixture of their two remaining cone populations, and this results in a narrower range of colour detection.

The absence of functional blue cones is called tritanopia, not tritanomaly. Both of these conditions are rare in comparison to red–green defects. The gene for blue (short-wavelength-sensitive) cones is on chromosome 7, whereas the genes for green and red cones are on the X chromosome.

106. D Somatomedins (e.g. IGF-1) result in decreased secretion of growth hormone

Pituitary adenomas may be functioning (resulting in over- or under-secretion of hormones) or non-functioning (no effect on hormone secretion).

Follicle-stimulating hormone is secreted by gonadotrophs in the anterior lobe of the pituitary gland.

The control of pituitary secretions involves hypothalamic hormones, peripheral circulating hormones and feedback loops. Short negative feedback loops occur from the action of pituitary hormones on the hypothalamus, whereas the secretions of peripheral endocrine glands result in long negative feedback loops. Examples of the latter include:

- Glucocorticoids, which exert negative feedback on the hypothalamus, reducing the secretion of corticotrophin-releasing factor (CRF)
- Somatomedins, such as insulin-like growth factor 1 (IGF-1), which are produced primarily by the liver and feed back to the hypothalamus to produce somatostatin, inhibiting the release of growth hormone, in addition to directly suppressing growth hormone secretion at the anterior pituitary

107. C Trigeminal nerve (V)

The oculocardiac reflex is trigemino–vagal: the afferent limb is the trigeminal nerve (V) and the efferent is the vagus nerve (X). Sensory fibres from the extraocular muscles travel via the long and short ciliary nerves to the ciliary ganglion (they do not synapse there), along the nasociliary nerve and then the ophthalmic division of the trigeminal nerve to the brainstem. The efferent limb is from the brainstem to the heart via the vagus nerve.

The oculocardiac reflex is elicited primarily by traction on the extraocular muscles, particularly the medial rectus. This typically occurs during squint surgery but may also occur in orbital fractures with muscle entrapment. It causes vagally-mediated sinus bradycardia, which may be severe enough to lead to asystole.

108. D The tension on the zonules increases

Contraction of the ciliary muscle, which is circular, decreases tension on the zonules, allowing the lens to thicken anteroposteriorly, resulting in an increase in its dioptric power. This is accompanied by other changes in the eye:

- The anterior pole moves forward with a slight increase in the axial length and decrease in equatorial diameter due to circumferential traction on the sclera
- The choroid is pulled anteriorly
- Aqueous outflow is increased via traction on the trabecular fibres (the outer longitudinal muscle fibres of the ciliary muscle attach directly to the scleral spur)

109. C The most common reason is inadequate dietary intake

Vitamin B12 (cobalamin) is a water-soluble vitamin whose deficiency causes neuropathy and anaemia. It is required as a cofactor by methionine synthase for the conversion of homocysteine to methionine. Homocysteine levels are therefore typically elevated in B12 deficiency.

Vitamin B12 deficiency can cause a painless, bilateral optic neuropathy that may precede anaemia. One of the most serious neurological manifestations is subacute combined degeneration of the spinal cord.

Dietary sources of vitamin B12 include eggs and meat. However, inadequate dietary intake is relatively rare compared to other causes. Gastric intrinsic factor is required for absorption of vitamin B12, which occurs in the terminal ileum. More common causes of vitamin B12 deficiency are (a) a lack of intrinsic factor due to pernicious anaemia or gastric resection, or (b) resection or disease of the terminal ileum.

110. B Osmolality refers to osmoles per litre of solution

If a salt, e.g. sodium chloride, dissociates in solution, then both sodium and chloride ions contribute to the osmotic pressure of the solution. Thus, 1 mole of a salt that dissociates entirely into two ions will give 2 osmoles of osmotic pressure. Osmoles are effectively the molecular weight of the solute divided by the number of ions/particles it dissociates into when in solution.

The number of osmoles:

- Per litre of solution = osmolarity
- Per kg of solvent = osmolality

These are often (incorrectly) used interchangeably, but proteins and lipids in plasma can lead to differences between the two measurements, as the total solvent weight (osmolality) does not include the weight of solutes, whereas the total volume (osmolarity) does include the solute volume. The osmolality of plasma is normally 280–305 mosmol/kg.

Osmoreceptors are found in the anterior hypothalamus, which is outside the blood-brain barrier, and can stimulate vasopressin (ADH) release in response to changes in osmolality.

111. C The principal secretory immunoglobulin in tears is IgG

The principal secretory immunoglobulin in tears is IgA. Tears as secreted by the lacrimal gland are isotonic with serum, although the concentrations of individual ions and proteins are different. The four principal tear proteins in lacrimal gland secretions are lysozyme, lactoferrin, lipocalcin and secretory IgA. A large number of other proteins have been reported in variable but smaller concentrations. These proteins have antimicrobial and supportive functions. Lysozyme is a protein that damages bacterial cell walls and has a significant antimicrobial effect.

112. A Conjunctival goblet cells

The ocular tear film is composed of three layers: an inner mucin layer secreted by the conjunctival goblet cells, an aqueous layer secreted by the glands of Wolfring, Krause's glands and (predominantly) the lacrimal gland, and an outer lipid layer secreted by the Meibomian glands. The mucin layer permits the aqueous layer to spread evenly across the otherwise hydrophobic epithelium of the cornea and conjunctiva. The lipid layer reduces evaporation of the aqueous layer.

113. D 99%

The vitreous, although a jelly-like substance, is composed of 98–99.7% water. The remaining mass comes almost entirely from collagen fibrils (composed of types II, V/XI and IX collagen) and glycosaminoglycans, predominantly hyaluronan.

114. D Uveoscleral outflow is largely independent of intraocular pressure

The trabecular route of aqueous outflow is pressure dependent, whereas the uveoscleral route is largely independent of intraocular pressure. The uveoscleral rate of drainage has previously been calculated as 0.3 μL/min. The percentage contribution of the uveoscleral flow to aqueous drainage varies; it is at least 10% and may be as high as 20–40%.

Aqueous drainage via the uveoscleral route passes via the suprachoroidal spaces into the choroidal circulation, whereas trabecular outflow drains into the episcleral veins. The trabecular meshwork has the highest resistance to flow at its outermost, juxtacanalicular zone.

115. C The cell bodies of the nerve fibres are found in the lateral geniculate nucleus

The cell bodies of the nerves of the optic radiations are located in the lateral geniculate nucleus. Fibres corresponding to the peripheral retina have a more widely looping course than those corresponding to the macula, which pass posteriorly in a more direct manner. Meyer's loop is a wide fan-shaped anterior loop which passes around the temporal horn of the lateral ventricle.

The parietal optic radiation carries information from the superior retina, and therefore information about the inferior visual field. Conversely the temporal optic radiation carries information from the inferior retina and therefore the superior visual field. This is important for understanding the effects of lesions involving these radiations.

116. A CSF has a lower chloride concentration than plasma

Under physiological conditions, compared to plasma, cerebrospinal fluid (CSF) has:
- Higher concentrations of chloride, magnesium and hydrogen ions
- Lower concentrations of glucose, protein, cholesterol
- Lower pH (~ 7.33)

Chloride, magnesium and hydrogen ions are outliers in CSF as they exist in higher concentrations than the plasma. Protein and cholesterol levels in normal CSF are extremely low.

117. B Parvocellular ganglions are predominantly found in the peripheral retina

The visual pathways from the retina to the brain are largely segregated into magnocellular and parvocellular pathways. A third pathway via neurons with extremely small cell bodies, called the koniocellular pathway, is less well characterised at present. The magnocellular pathway is a 'coarse-grained' motion-sensitive pathway originating principally in the peripheral retina, and the parvocellular pathway is a 'fine-grained' high detail pathway that dominates at the fovea. The key differences between the two pathways are summarised in Table 2.11.

Table 2.11 Key differences between magnocellular and parvocellular pathways	
Magnocellular pathway	Parvocellular pathway
Ganglions have larger cell body	Ganglions have smaller cell body
Ganglions have large receptive field	Ganglions have small receptive field
Predominantly from peripheral retina	Predominantly from fovea
Project to layers 1 and 2 of lateral geniculate nucleus (LGN)	Project to layers 3–6 of LGN
Terminates primarily in layer 4Cα of V1	Terminates primarily in layer 4Cβ of V1
High contrast sensitivity	Lower contrast sensitivity
More sensitive to movement	More sensitive to form
Insensitive to colour	Sensitive to colour
Responses are transient	Responses are sustained

Statistics and evidence-based medicine

118. A 10%

Absolute risk reduction is the absolute difference between the percentage of patients experiencing an outcome in the treatment group and those experiencing the outcome in another group (in this case in a placebo group). Thus:

$$20\% - (2 \times 5)\% = 10\% \text{ absolute risk reduction}$$

It is important to know the difference between this and relative risk reduction, which is the absolute risk reduction expressed as a percentage of the non-treatment risk. In the case of this example it would be calculated as:

$$\frac{10}{20} \times 100 = 50\% \text{ relative risk reduction}$$

119. C III

Phase III clinical trials, testing a drug's effectiveness against the current gold standard treatment, are required in order to be granted a marketing licence.

To be allowed to progress to a phase III trial, the drug must first have gone through successful phase I and II trials. These establish safety, dosing and efficacy in the target population.

Phase IV trials are not compulsory and are performed once the drug is on the market.

These phases are outlined in Table 3.2 (page 207).

120. B χ^2

Of the options given, only the χ^2 test is a non-parametric test. This means that no assumptions are made about the defining parameters of the population. Parametric tests, by contrast, assume a normal distribution of the population. A normally-distributed population is defined by specific parameters, e.g. the mean, standard deviation, and variance. It is therefore not always possible to apply parametric tests.

Examples of parametric tests include Student's t test, the z test, Pearson's test, and analysis of variance (ANOVA). Examples of non-parametric tests include the χ^2 test, Fisher's exact test, and the Mann–Whitney (Wilcoxon rank sum) test.

If there is a difference between two populations, it is more likely to be discovered using parametric tests.

Answers: CRQs

Anatomy

1. Answer

(a)

    A – Schwalbe's line

    B – Trabecular meshwork

    C – Scleral spur

    D – Ciliary body

    (1 mark for each correctly named structure)

(b) Aqueous humour passes from the anterior chamber through the trabecular meshwork (intertrabecular and intratrabecular spaces) and into Schlemm's canal. From Schlemm's canal the aqueous drains through collector channels and the aqueous veins of Ascher into venous plexuses, and conjunctival and episcleral veins
(1 mark for each stage:
- *Trabecular meshwork to Schlemm's canal*
- *Schlemm's canal to collector channels and aqueous veins (of Ascher)*
- *Collector channels and aqueous veins of Ascher to venous plexuses and conjunctival veins)*

(c) A rise in intraocular pressure has no effect (or a minimal effect) on the drainage via the non-conventional (uveoscleral) pathway, as this pathway is not pressure sensitive.

Feedback
Sensitivity to intraocular pressure is one of the key differences between the behaviour of the conventional and non-conventional (uveoscleral) outflow pathways. The non-conventional pathway is not sensitive to fluctuations in intraocular pressure, whereas the conventional pathway is pressure-sensitive and modulates outflow resistance to regulate intraocular pressure.

(d) Pilocarpine stimulates contraction of the sphincter pupillae and the ciliary muscle via muscarinic receptors. This opens the trabecular meshwork, increasing outflow via the conventional pathway.

(e) Prostaglandin analogues

Feedback
The key mechanisms of action of different classes of glaucoma medications are summarised in **Table 2.12**.

Table 2.12 Mechanisms of action of glaucoma medications	
Medication class	Mechanism of action
Prostaglandin analogues (e.g. latanoprost)	Increased uveoscleral outflow
Beta-blockers (e.g. timolol)	Decreased aqueous humour production
$α_2$-adrenergic agonists (e.g. brimonidine)	Decreased aqueous production and increased outflow at least partially via the uveoscleral pathway
Carbonic anhydrase inhibitors (e.g. dorzolamide)	Decreased aqueous production
Parasympathomimetics (e.g. pilocarpine)	Increased outflow via conventional pathway
Hyperosmotic agents (e.g. mannitol)	Decreased vitreous volume

Pharmacology

2. Answer

(a) G-protein-coupled receptor (metabotropic receptor also acceptable)

Feedback
G-protein-coupled receptors, which are metabotropic (as opposed to ionotropic) receptors, have seven transmembrane domains with an intracellular binding site for a G protein. The G protein itself is membrane-bound and composed of three subunits.

(b)

W – Transmembrane domain of G-protein-coupled receptor (GPCR)

X – G protein binding site of GPCR

Y – G protein α subunit

Z – G protein βγ subunits

(½ mark for each correct label)

(c) Rhodopsin is a G-protein-coupled receptor found in the outer segments of rod photoreceptors. It is activated not by ligand binding, but by light-activated isomerisation of prebound 11-*cis*-retinal to all-*trans*-retinal. The process triggered by activation of rhodopsin is phototransduction, which converts light energy into an electrical signal. Activation of the receptor causes binding and activation of the G protein, transducin, with signal transduction via cGMP phosphodiesterase resulting in the closure of cGMP-gated cation channels. This causes hyperpolarisation of the photoreceptor cell, which modulates neurotransmitter release at the synapse with bipolar cells.

(1 mark each for: naming the receptor, describing activation, naming phototransduction, describing briefly the process of phototransduction)

(d)
- Beta-blockers/β adrenoreceptor antagonists
- α_2 adrenoreceptor agonists
- Muscarinic ACh receptor agonists/cholinergics

Feedback
G-protein-coupled receptors (GPCRs) are common drug targets and glaucoma medication is no exception. Three of the common classes of intraocular pressure-lowering agents are either agonists or antagonists at GPCRs. They influence intraocular pressure (IOP) via their effects on the autonomic innervation of the eye. Their resulting effects on aqueous production and outflow are described in **Table 2.12** above.

Investigations and imaging

3. Answer

(a) Static automated perimetry

Feedback
Humphrey perimetry (visual field testing) is a static, automated visual field test. 'Static' refers to the presentation of visual stimuli: these are stationary, but presented at differing intensities and at different points throughout the potential visual field to determine the sensitivity of the eye at each point. This differs from kinetic perimetry, where the stimulus is a moving target of a set luminance.

Perimetry may be automated or manual, the latter involving an operator choosing when and where to present each stimulus. The Humphrey field analyser is a commonly-used static, automated perimeter; whereas Goldmann perimetry is a good example of a kinetic perimeter, which can be manual or automated (it is classically a kinetic test, but may also be used as a static test for the central field).

In manual perimetry, the operator can adapt the speed of the test to the patient. Furthermore, it can be useful in supporting a diagnosis of non-organic field loss, e.g. demonstrating spiralling of the visual field and crossing of isoptres. However, static automated perimetry has many advantages, being a standardised test that is better at detecting and mapping relative scotomas, as well as performing statistical analysis.

(b) This is a reliable test. The fixation losses, false positive and false negative error rates are all very low.
(*1 mark for reliability; 1 mark for reasoning*)

Feedback
The fixation losses, false negative and false positive rates together provide useful information on the reliability of the test. Fixation losses or false negatives of >20%

may compromise the reliability of the test. False negative rates may represent fatigue or poor concentration, and are recorded when a point correctly seen by a patient is not seen on a retest with a brighter stimulus. False positives indicate 'trigger happy' patients who press the button with no stimulus, and should ideally be <10%.

(c) The pattern standard deviation (PSD) is a measure of the patient's overall deviation that is adjusted for generalised depression in the visual field (i.e. the deviation of a given area relative to the rest of the patient's field).

Feedback
Whereas mean deviation (MD) simply measures the patient's values for each data point in the field compared to age-matched norms, the PSD is useful as it is adjusted for generalised depression of the field. Generalised depression represents diffuse visual loss throughout the field, commonly due to cataract. Thus, the PSD would be more useful for detecting glaucomatous field loss in a patient with cataract than the MD.

(d) The differential intensity of the light stimulus is graded on a logarithmic scale (*1 mark*). The stimulus is varied by placing neutral density filters of different strengths, graded in decibels, over a maximally-emitting light bulb (*1 mark*)

Feedback
The luminance of the background and the stimulus must be carefully controlled in visual field testing.

The background luminance is kept constant and is measured in apostilbs (asb). One apostilb is equivalent to 1 lumen per square metre (or $1/\pi$ candela per square metre). The Humphrey perimeter has a background luminance of 31.5 asb, and a stimulus light with a maximal luminance of 10,000 asb. To vary the intensity of the stimulus, neutral density filters are interposed and these are graded in decibels (dB). Decibels are logarithmic units to the base 10. They do not exclusively apply to sound.

The numerical display at the top left of the page in the figures (page 112 and 113) shows the sensitivities at different points in the visual field: the higher the number, the higher the optical density of the filter in front of the light bulb, and thus the dimmer the stimulus used. A point of 0 dB means that the stimulus was maximal intensity (10,000 asb). The dimmest stimulus this patient detected was 33 dB (right eye).

(e) Left inferior arcuate/altitudinal field defect

(f) Left optic nerve

Feedback
This patient has a unilateral arcuate or altitudinal defect that suggests left optic nerve pathology.

(g)
- Glaucoma
- Ischaemic optic neuropathy
- Hemiretinal (or branch) artery or vein occlusion (superior)
- Optic neuritis
- Compressive optic nerve lesion
  (*1 mark each up to 2 marks*)

Feedback
These fields were performed by a patient with advanced unilateral primary open angle glaucoma. The patient presented with bilateral high intraocular pressures, at a point where glaucomatous damage had occurred in the left but not the right eye. The fields supported but did not make the diagnosis. Especially with unilateral glaucomatous field loss, there is an important differential including compressive lesions.

4. Answer

(a) Systemic lupus erythematosus (SLE)

Feedback
The non-ocular clinical features in this case are arthritis, mouth ulcers, lethargy and a photosensitive rash. Although all consistent with SLE, they are non-specific, and the laboratory tests are required to help make the diagnosis in this case.

The commonest aetiology of retinal vein occlusions is atherosclerosis, with hypertension being an important risk factor. The ocular finding of a central retinal vein occlusion is slightly unusual in a middle-aged patient with no cardiovascular risk factors, prompting investigations to look for any underlying vasculitis or haematological cause.

The blood test abnormalities in this case, many of which are mild, are lymphopenia, thrombocytopenia, raised erythrocyte sedimentation rate (ESR), positive antinuclear antibodies (ANA) and elevated IgG immunoglobulins. This constellation of results is consistent with SLE. A raised ESR tends to be accompanied by a normal C-reactive protein (CRP) in SLE, unless the patient has, for example, active synovitis. The combination of normal CRP and raised ESR in a multisystem disorder should raise suspicion of SLE, although it can also be seen in other inflammatory processes. Immunoglobulins are elevated due to the production of autoantibodies, which subsequently form immune complexes that are deposited in tissues.

(b) Autoantibodies, including:
- Anti-double-stranded DNA (anti-dsDNA)
- Extractable nuclear antigen (ENA) antibodies (anti-Ro or anti-La)
- Anti-Smith antibodies
- Antiphospholipid antibodies (lupus anticoagulant, anticardiolipin, anti-β2 glycoprotein)
  (*1 mark for either autoantibodies or any of the specific tests listed*)

Feedback
Anti-ds DNA is highly specific for systemic lupus erythematosus (SLE) and has a sensitivity of 60–70%. By contrast, antinuclear antibody (ANA) has a sensitivity of 95% but is not specific. A wide range of autoantibodies may be positive in SLE, reflecting the cellular components that are targeted by the immune hypersensitivity reaction.

Antiphospholipid antibodies may occur in SLE and include lupus anticoagulant and anticardiolipin. Lupus anticoagulant is to some extent a misnomer. Whilst in vitro it has anticoagulant properties, the presence of this autoantibody in vivo is procoagulant. Furthermore, it is not specific to SLE but is also found in antiphospholipid syndrome due to other causes.

(c) Any two of:
- Dry eyes
- Central or branch retinal artery occlusion
- Vaso-occlusive retinopathy
- Optic neuropathy
- Anterior uveitis
- Episcleritis
- Scleritis
- Keratitis
- Myositis (of extraocular muscles)
- Choroidal effusion and/or exudative retinal detachment
- Orbital vasculitis
- Eyelid/orbital panniculitis
- Discoid lupus of the eyelids

Feedback
Systemic lupus erythematosus can affect almost any structure within the eye either through inflammation or vascular occlusion. Whilst not part of the diagnostic criteria, ophthalmic manifestations are common. Orbital involvement is rare.

(d) Polyclonal. Paraproteins were not detected on protein electrophoresis.

(1 mark for polyclonal; 1 mark for reasoning)

Feedback
If the rise in immunoglobulins was monoclonal, a paraprotein band would typically be seen on protein electrophoresis. This would suggest myeloma or other monoclonal gammopathy. The protein electrophoresis in this case did not detect a paraprotein band. Causes of a polyclonal rise in immunoglobulins include infections, chronic liver disease and autoimmune diseases such as systemic lupus erythematosus and rheumatoid arthritis.

(e) Systemic lupus erythematosus may cause retinal vein occlusion via phlebitis of the retinal veins or via a prothrombotic tendency caused by antiphospholipid syndrome.
(1 mark for each mechanism)

(f) Any two of:
- Cystoid macular oedema
- Neovascularisation (rubeosis)
- Vitreous haemorrhage
- Neovascular/rubeotic glaucoma
- Epiretinal membrane

Feedback
Cystoid macular oedema (CMO) can occur in both ischaemic and non-ischaemic central retinal vein occlusion (CRVO). Its presence may be confirmed on optical coherence tomography (most common modality) or fundus fluorescein angiography (FFA). It is an indication for intravitreal treatment with anti-vascular endothelial growth factor (anti-VEGF) or steroids.

Neovascularisation can occur in ischaemic CRVO, and new vessels are seen at the iris, disc or elsewhere in the retina (usually in that order). New vessels show a typical leakage pattern on FFA, and may bleed to cause vitreous haemorrhage. Treatment may include panretinal photocoagulation and anti-VEGF, and vitrectomy if required for vitreous haemorrhage. Neovascular glaucoma is due to new vessels in the drainage angle which eventually cause synechial closure of the angle. Treatment is directed at controlling neovascularisation, intraocular pressure, inflammation and pain.

5. Answer

(a) Hydrogen atoms or protons *(1 mark for either nomenclature)*

Feedback
During MRI a strong static magnetic field causes the protons in the body to align along the direction of the magnetic field. In this state they rotate (precess) around their own axes in different phases. A radiofrequency (RF) pulse is applied, tuned to a specific frequency range. This transfers energy to the protons, altering the alignment of some of them and causing them to precess in phase with each other. As the RF pulse dissipates the protons lose energy, start to realign along the original (static) magnetic field (T1 relaxation) and begin to precess out of phase (T2 relaxation). The relaxation of protons releases weak RF signals (called echo) which are detected by receiver coils and used in the computerised construction of the images.

(b) T2-weighted

Feedback
In an MRI of the head the easiest way to differentiate between T1-weighted and T2-weighted pulse sequences is the colour of low-protein fluid such as the cerebrospinal fluid (e.g. in the ventricles) or the vitreous. In T1-weighted images this will be black, whereas in T2-weighted images this will be lighter (often essentially white). For a summary of the different characteristics of T1-weighted and T2-weighted images please see Table 1.5 on page 46.

(c) Any four of:

- No ionising radiation
- High soft tissue contrast
- Potential to image vasculature without contrast
- No artefact from bone (advantageous in posterior fossa imaging)
- Option of tissue-targeted modification of images (e.g. STIR fat suppression)
- Potential to perform functional imaging (e.g. diffusion-weighted imaging, DWI) and measure blood flow (functional MRI)
- Potential to produce multiplanar images without having to reposition the patient

(1 mark for each up to 4 marks. Only include 4 answers)

Feedback
The absence of ionising radiation means that MRI can be undertaken with confidence on pregnant and paediatric patients. It provides high soft tissue contrast relative to CT (e.g. differentiating grey and white matter) and it is possible to image the major vasculature without administering contrast (useful in patients with a history of contrast reactions or those at risk of contrast-induced nephropathy). There is no bone artefact.

Fat suppression imaging has a number of applications, including the assessment of active inflammation in thyroid eye disease.

Diffusion-weighted imaging assesses the movement of water molecules and can be used to help characterise abnormalities (e.g. acute ischaemic infarcts show restricted diffusion).

Functional MRI (fMRI) can be used to map changes in metabolic rate (and therefore indirectly neural activity) by measuring the change in magnetisation between blood of different oxygen concentrations. To date it has mostly been used in a research setting.

Finally, MRI can produce multiplanar images (axial, coronal and sagittal/parasagittal) without needing to reposition the patient, whereas CT scans traditionally acquire images in the axial plane. Modern CT scanners are now able to reconstruct images in multiple planes with good spatial resolution, so this advantage only applies when comparing MRI to older CT machines.

(d) Midline shift (or subfalcine herniation); sulcal effacement; ventricular effacement.
(1 mark for each. ½ mark if displacement of brain parenchyma is given instead of midline shift)

Feedback
This image shows pronounced midline shift to the left (with anterior subfalcine herniation) and effacement of the cortical sulci in the right frontal lobe. There is effacement of the right lateral ventricle (the left ventricle also appears effaced in this section, although in fact it is displaced and slightly enlarged). Note that the large right anterior mass is not in itself a sign of mass effect.

(e) VI (abducens) nerve palsy due to raised intracranial pressure

Feedback
Neurological signs are described as 'false-localising' if they represent a functional change based on an anatomical locus that is different from the site of the primary pathology. With raised intracranial pressure the most common false localising sign is VI (abducens) nerve palsy, which may be unilateral or bilateral. The most commonly given explanation for this is that it is due to the stretching of the nerve during its long intracranial course where it is relatively tethered in Dorello's canal.

6. Answer

(a) Amsler chart, or Amsler grid *(1 mark if either term used)*

Feedback
An Amsler chart is a regular grid of squares with a fixation spot in the middle. Some versions have white lines on a dark background. There are a number of modified Amsler charts available.

(b) The patient tests one eye at a time by covering or closing the other eye. With the open eye they focus on the dark spot in the centre of the grid. They should wear their normal reading glasses if they usually need these and hold the chart at 30–35 cm (12–14 in). In a healthy macula the grid should appear regular and complete – an abnormal result is one in which the lines are distorted, blurred or have sections missing.
(1 mark each for:

- *Occluding other eye to make test monocular*
- *Focussing on the spot at the centre of the grid*
- *Normal reading glasses*
- *Appropriate distance; normal reading distance also acceptable*
- *What constitutes an abnormal result)*

Feedback
The key points in this explanation are highlighted above under the mark scheme. It is important to be able to give a clear, succinct explanation of how to conduct such tests as you may be under time pressure in the examination.

(c) To guide the patient's gaze to the fixation point

Feedback
This type of Amsler chart is particularly useful in patients with a significant central scotoma, who find fixation on a small point extremely difficult.

(d) You should look at everyday objects which you know are straight, such as the edge of doors, bathroom tiles, the edge of television screens, photo frames, railings, and see if they are becoming more distorted or blurred in either eye (closing the other eye). You should also monitor your reading ability and overall image quality. You can wear your normal distance and reading glasses.

(1 mark each for:

- Monitoring using everyday objects with a straight edge
- Monocular testing
- Wearing normal distance and reading glasses)

Feedback
So called 'environmental Amsler' testing has been shown, with appropriate patient selection and training, to have a high sensitivity and specificity for predicting which patients undergoing anti-vascular endothelial growth factor injections require further treatment. It is important to be able to explain to patients how to use their own environment to monitor their condition.

Microbiology

7. Answer

(a) Crystal violet dye is applied to the specimen which stains peptidoglycans in the cell walls of Gram positive bacteria. Iodine is then applied, which fixes crystal violet to the cells it has stained. The specimen is then washed with either acetone or ethanol to remove the remaining crystal violet and iodine. Finally a counterstain is applied (usually safranin, although sometimes fuchsine is used) which allows visualisation of Gram negative bacteria.

(1 mark for the crystal violet primary stain; 1 mark for describing binding to the cell walls of Gram positive bacteria; 1 mark for iodine fixing; 1 mark for washout; 1 mark for counterstain to show Gram negative bacteria; specific name of counterstain not required)

Feedback
The Gram stain is one of the most fundamental diagnostic techniques in microbiology and it is helpful to understand its basic principles. With this technique Gram positive organisms are stained a purple colour, whereas Gram negative organisms are stained a pink/red by the counterstain.

(b) *Haemophilus influenzae* and *Pseudomonas aeruginosa* (1 mark for each – ½ mark if *Moraxella* species given in place of either)

Feedback
In the Western world the majority of organisms identified in cases of post-operative endophthalmitis are Gram positive (in particular coagulase-negative staphylococci, *Staphylococcus aureus*, β-haemolytic streptococci and *Enterococcus faecalis*). However, the organisms in this case are staining pink/red with the counterstain and are therefore Gram negative. The two most common Gram negative organisms in acute endophthalmitis in the Western world are *Haemophilus influenzae* and *Pseudomonas aeruginosa*, both of which are coccobacilli. *Moraxella species* when grouped together provide the third most common Gram negative cause. A higher

proportion of endophthalmitis cases are secondary to Gram negative organisms in India and China. Additionally, endogenous endophthalmitis may be secondary to Gram negative organisms such as *Escherichia coli*, *Neisseria meningitidis*, and *Klebsiella species*.

(c) Neutrophils

Feedback
Neutrophils are the principal component of the initial immune cellular infiltrate. They release lytic enzymes which cause extensive destruction in all layers of the retina. As the inflammation enters the acceleration phase there is typically increased recruitment of macrophages and lymphocytes into the vitreous cavity.

(d) Amikacin

Feedback
Amikacin (an aminoglycoside) has good activity against Gram negative organisms and is commonly utilised for intravitreal injection. It is particularly useful in patients with a significant penicillin allergy, where cephalosporins, such as ceftazidime, are contraindicated for intravitreal injection. Gentamicin is also sometimes used for Gram negative cover, and is also an acceptable answer to this question, but there have been concerns regarding retinal toxicity. Vancomycin is usually also administered to cover Gram positive organisms.

(e) Amikacin has poor penetration into the vitreous from the circulation

Feedback
It is important to be aware of the tissue penetration of antibiotics when considering administration routes. Amikacin and ceftazidime have poor ocular penetration, and intravenous administration of these agents does not improve outcome in endophthalmitis. Conversely fluoroquinolones, such as ciprofloxacin, have much better tissue penetration, including in the eye, and systemic treatment with these agents may be a useful adjunct to intravitreal therapy.

Pathology

8. Answer

(a) The figures show ocular ultrasound:
- Figure a: B-scan ultrasound
- Figure b: A-scan ultrasound

(½ mark for ultrasound, ½ mark for A- and B-scan)

(b) Ultrasound is based on the principle of acoustic impedance. A piezoelectric crystal transducer converts electrical energy into high-frequency sound waves which travel through the tissues. The reflected signal (echo) from the target tissue is detected by the transducer and its magnitude measured.

Echoes are generated from the interface of tissues with different acoustic impedance. Higher frequencies give greater resolution but less depth of penetration.

A-scan ultrasound plots the intensity of the echo versus time delay, which can be converted into distance based on the speed of sound in the tissue. B-scan images are two-dimensional and generated from multiple transverse A-scans.

(1 mark each for including: high-frequency sound waves; echo from target tissue; A-scan versus B-scan description)

Feedback
Ultrasound waves have a frequency higher than the audible range for humans (≥20,000 Hz, or 20 kHz). The frequencies used in medical ultrasound are typically 8–100 MHz.

A reflected sound wave is transduced back into an electrical signal by the piezoelectric transducer and amplified. The degree of amplification, the 'gain', can be adjusted depending on the structure of interest. As the echo is generated from a change in the impedance of a tissue, if a tissue is very homogeneous then no signal will be reflected.

A-scan and B-scan ultrasound are often used concurrently, as in the images shown.

(c) The B-scan shows a large, solid lesion at the posterior pole of the eye that seems to be arising from the choroid and is collar-stud or mushroom-shaped in appearance. There is an associated retinal detachment. The lesion has low internal reflectivity on A-scan ultrasound.

(1 mark for large/solid lesion, 1 mark for collar-stud/mushroom-shaped, 1 mark for low internal reflectivity, 1 mark for retinal detachment. Maximum 2 marks)

(d) Choroidal melanoma

Feedback
This is a typical appearance for a choroidal melanoma. They appear as solid lesions arising from the choroid which typically have low to medium internal reflectivity. Sometimes choroidal excavation is evident. The appearance of the tumour is often dome-shaped, but a characteristic mushroom or collar-stud appearance such as this occurs in 20% of cases due to rupture through Bruch's membrane.

(e)
- Large size
- Extrascleral extension
- Epithelioid cell type
- High mitotic count
- Monosomy 3

- Duplication of 8q
- Closed loop vascular pattern on periodic acid–Schiff (PAS) stain

(1 mark for each correct prognostic factor up to 3 marks)

Feedback
In addition to the histopathological and cytogenetic factors listed above, older age is also associated with a worse prognosis.

Histological examination of choroidal melanomas allows classification by cell type: epithelioid, spindle, or mixed. Epithelioid cell-containing tumours carry a worse prognosis. Immunohistochemistry can help to confirm the diagnosis, with tumours tending to stain positive for S100, melan-A and HMB-45.

Cytogenetics are extremely valuable prognostically, as metastatic death occurs almost solely in patients with choroidal melanomas with loss of chromosome 3. Mortality is worse with both loss of chromosome 3 and gain of 8q.

Optics

9. Answer

(a)

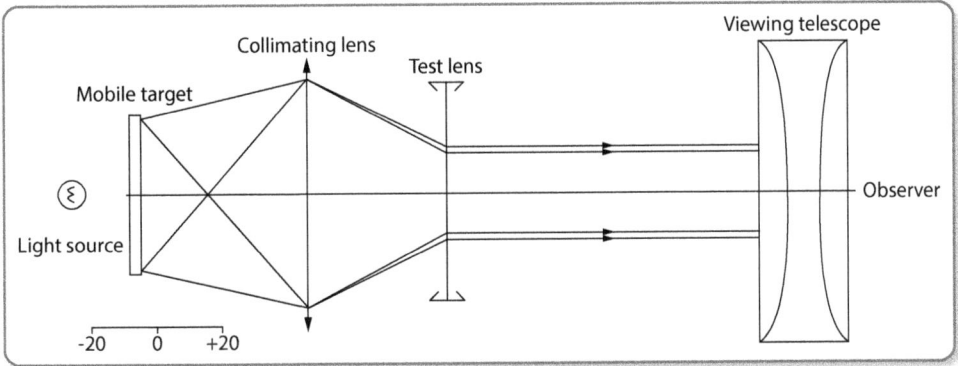

Feedback
The key components of this ray diagram are the light source and target *(1 mark)*, collimating lens *(1 mark)*, test lens (positioned at the principal focus of the collimating lens) *(1 mark)* and the parallel rays emerging from the test lens and continuing to the viewing telescope once the instrument is focussed *(1 mark)*.

(b) Glasses should be oriented so that their back surface is facing the light source and collimating lens (and therefore their front surface is facing the user). This is because spectacles are prescribed according to their back vertex power, and therefore this is the power that should be measured.

(c) +1.00 DS/ +2.00 DC at 30° (plus cylinder format)

+3.00 DS/ −2.00 DC at 120° (minus cylinder format)

(1 mark each for sphere, cylinder and axis)

Feedback
If choosing plus cylinder format, you should take the least plus (most minus) power as your base sphere and add the difference in the two powers as your cylinder with the axis shown at the most plus (least minus) power.

If choosing minus cylinder format, you should take the most plus (least minus) power as your base sphere and subtract the difference in the two powers as your cylinder with the axis shown at the least plus (most minus) power.

(d) This lens is a concave (minus) lens without any astigmatic correction (cylinder)

Feedback
Concave lenses cause the image of the cross to move in the same direction as the lens (a 'with' movement) whilst convex (plus) lenses cause the image of the cross to move in the opposite direction (an 'against' movement). We know the lens does not have any astigmatic correction (i.e. it is spherical) as there is no scissoring of the cross on rotation of the lens.

(e) This lens has a base up prism incorporated.

Feedback
Prisms will always displace one line of the cross regardless of lens position, as a prism has no optical centre. The image is displaced towards the apex of the prism and therefore the base is in the opposite direction to the displaced image.

- Base up: image displaced downwards
- Base down: image displaced upwards
- Base in: image displaced outwards
- Base out: image displaced inwards

10. Answer

(a) The pathogenesis of dry AMD is characterised by:

- Degeneration of the retinal pigment epithelium
- Loss of photoreceptors
- Accumulation of lipofuscin
- Drusen formation
- Thickening of Bruch's membrane
- Thinning of the outer plexiform layer and choriocapillaris

(1 mark each up to 2 marks)

(b) Magnifiers present an enlarged retinal image by increasing the angle subtended by the object at the eye.

(c)

Convex lens acting as a magnifier

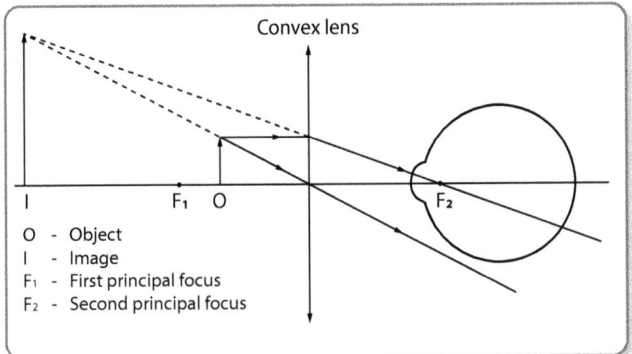

(3 marks for diagram including convex lens, object within principal focus of lens, and either magnified image or increase in angle subtended at the eye)

(d)

Diagram of a Galilean telescope

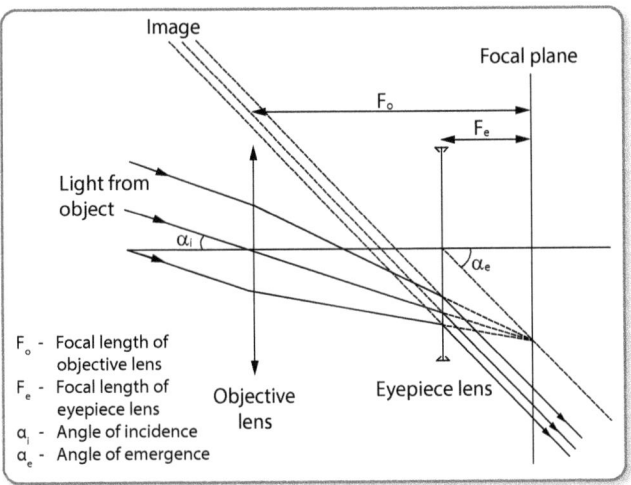

(1 mark each for including: convex objective lens, concave eyepiece lens, lenses in correct position, parallel incident and emergent rays)

11. Answer

(a) Light Amplification by the Stimulated Emission of Radiation

(b) Laser beams are typically coherent, collimated and monochromatic *(1 mark each)*. Another way of phrasing this is that the rays of light are in phase, parallel and all of the same wavelength

(c)

Laser beam production

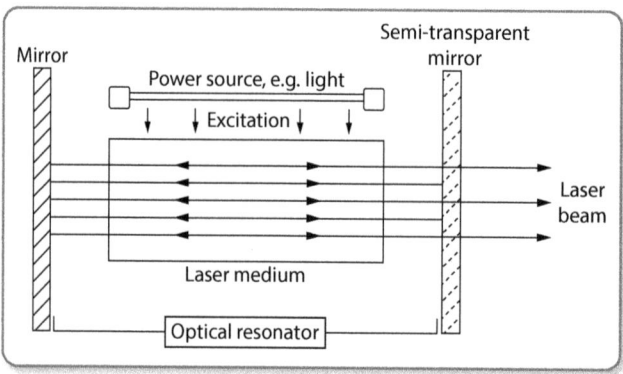

(1 mark each for power source, laser medium, semi-transparent mirror, and rays)

(d) Any two of:
- Argon laser: The active medium is argon blue–green gas; used for panretinal photocoagulation (PRP), laser retinopexy, focal/grid macular laser, and laser trabeculoplasty
- ND:YAG LASER: The active medium is neodymium–yttrium–aluminium–garnet; used for posterior (and anterior) capsulotomy, peripheral iridotomy and selective laser trabeculoplasty (SLT)
- The frequency-doubled Nd:YAG laser: Similar photocoagulation effect and indications as the argon laser
- Cyclodiode laser: The active medium is a diode chip; used trans-scerally to destroy the ciliary body to reduce intraocular pressure

(1 mark per laser up to two marks – must have correct medium and at least one correct procedure)

Feedback
The lasers above are all commonly used in the ophthalmology outpatient setting. Lasers used in corneal and refractive surgery, such as the excimer or femtosecond lasers, are excluded from this question as they can have a range of active laser media.

Statistics and evidence-based medicine

12. Answer

Please note, although some of these questions permit a calculator and are included here for practice, a calculator may not be required or permitted in the examination itself. Check examination guidelines in advance.

(a) 10%

Feedback
Labelling the results (as presented in **Table 2.13**) facilitates further calculations.

The false positive rate is calculated as the number of false positive cases divided by the total number of negative cases (regardless of how they were classified). In this question, the total number of patients without the disease is given, but for any situation the false positive rate can be calculated using the following equation:

$$FPR = \frac{FP}{FP + TN}$$

Where FPR is false positive rate, FP is the absolute number of false positives and TN is the absolute number of true negatives.

Table 2.13 Categorising results

	Disease present	Disease absent
Test positive	True positive (950)	False positive (100)
Test negative	False negative (50)	True negative (900)
Total	1,000 patients	1,000 patients

(b) Sensitivity = 950/(950 + 50) = 0.95 = 95%

Specificity = 900/(900 + 100) = 0.9 = 90%

Feedback
Sensitivity is the probability of a test being positive in those who have the disease. Specificity is the probability of a test being negative in those unaffected by the disease. **Table 2.14** shows how they are calculated. Neither of these measures are affected by the prevalence of the disease in the population.

Table 2.14 Sensitivity and specificity

	Disease present	Disease absent
Test positive	True positive (TP)	False positive (FP)
Test negative	False negative (FN)	True negative (TN)
	Sensitivity = $\frac{TP}{TP + FN}$	Specificity = $\frac{TN}{TN + FP}$

(c) Positive predictive value = 950/(950 + 100) = 0.905 = 90.5%

Negative predictive value = 900/(900 + 50) = 0.947 = 94.7%

Feedback
The positive predictive value (PPV) is the percentage of patients who test positive who truly have the disease. **Table 2.15** shows how it is calculated. The negative predictive value (NPV) is the percentage of patients who test negative who are truly negative. The predictive values are useful for determining the significance of a test result for an individual patient in that population. A high PPV makes the test useful for confirming a diagnosis, whereas a high NPV makes the test useful for excluding it. PPV and NPV are both dependent on the prevalence of the disease in a population. This is because the predictive values are calculated based on the total number of patients testing positive or negative, rather than grouping by whether the disease is present or absent (as in sensitivity and specificity).

When revising the difference between sensitivity/specificity and the predictive values, remember the denominator: for the former, the denominator is the presence/absence of disease, whereas for predictive values, the denominator is the test result.

Table 2.15 Positive and negative predictive values

	Disease present	Disease absent	Predictive values
Test positive	True positive (TP)	False positive (FP)	Positive predictive value $= \dfrac{TP}{TP + FP}$
Test negative	False negative (FN)	True negative (TN)	Negative predictive value $= \dfrac{TN}{TN + FN}$
Sensitivity/ Specificity	Sensitivity $= \dfrac{TP}{TP + FN}$	Specificity $= \dfrac{TN}{TN + FP}$	

(d) A positive test result is more useful in Marseille. As the prevalence of the disease in a population increases, the positive predictive value increases (assuming other factors remain constant). Therefore, for an individual patient with a positive test, the likelihood of them having glaucoma is higher in Marseille than in Birmingham.

(1 mark for correct city and 2 marks for explanation (PPV increasing as prevalence increases; implication for the individual patient), or for showing calculations of PPV in each population with explanation of implication for the individual patient)

Feedback
Unlike sensitivity and specificity, the predictive values are affected by the prevalence of the disease in the population. Assuming other factors remain constant, the positive predictive value (PPV) increases with increasing prevalence, whereas negative predictive value (NPV) decreases.

We have already calculated the sensitivity and specificity of this test and know the prevalence of glaucoma in each population. We can therefore calculate the PPV for each population as shown in **Tables 2.16** and **2.17**.

Table 2.16 Positive predictive value (PPV) for Birmingham

	Glaucoma patients	Patients without glaucoma	Predictive values
Test positive	9,500	99,000	Positive predictive value $= \dfrac{9,500}{9,500 + 99,000}$ $= \dfrac{9,500}{108,500}$ $= 8.8\%$
Test negative	500	891,000	
Total	10,000 patients	990,000 patients	

Table 2.17 Positive predictive value (PPV) for Marseille

	Glaucoma patients	Patients without glaucoma	Predictive values
Test positive	95,000	90,000	Positive predictive value $= \dfrac{95,000}{95,000 + 90,000}$ $= \dfrac{95,000}{185,500}$ $= 51.3\%$
Test negative	5,000	810,000	
Total	100,000 patients	900,000 patients	

The PPV of this test in Birmingham is 8.8% and the PPV in Marseille is 51.3%. Therefore, a positive test is more useful for predicting disease in a citizen of Marseille. In the original study 'population' in the question stem, two groups of equal size were compared and so the prevalence was in effect 50%, which gave a PPV of 90.5%.

(e) Any two of:
- Diabetic retinopathy
- Retinopathy of prematurity
- Amblyopia, strabismus and refractive errors in children

Feedback
There is a systematic, national screening programme for diabetic retinopathy in the UK. This involves digital fundus photography of all patients with diabetes, with standardised grading of images and strict criteria for referral to the hospital eye service.

Retinopathy of prematurity is also screened for systematically throughout the UK following national guidelines, which recommend screening for all babies born <32 weeks' gestation or <1,501 g birth weight, and mandate screening for all babies <31 weeks' gestation or <1,251 g birth weight.

Preschool or school-entry visual screening is also in place in the UK to detect amblyopia, refractive errors and strabismus.

Whilst other conditions are routinely screened for by optometrists, this is not a systematic screening programme applying to a whole subgroup of the population, as in the examples above.

Chapter 3

Exam Paper 3: Unstructured Mock Exam

Questions: SBAs

120 SBAs to be answered in 3 hours

For each question, please select the single best answer.

1. From which embryological cell population does the trabecular meshwork originate?

    A Mesoderm
    B Neural crest mesenchyme
    C Neuroectoderm
    D Surface ectoderm

2. An image produced by a concave mirror is real, inverted, enlarged and lies outside the centre of curvature. Where does the object lie?

    A At the principal focus
    B Between the centre of curvature and the principal focus
    C Between the principal focus and the mirror
    D Outside the centre of curvature

3. Which of the following antibiotics is least effective against Gram negative organisms?

    A Amoxicillin
    B Cefuroxime
    C Metronidazole
    D Vancomycin

4. Which of the following terms best describes a substance which only allows the transmission of light in an incident plane aligned with its structure, by absorbing other light waves?

    A Birefringent
    B Dichroic

C Mirrored
D Scattering

5. How far posterior to the limbus does the lateral rectus insert?
   A 5.5 mm
   B 6.5 mm
   C 6.9 mm
   D 7.7 mm

6. In which phase of clinical trial is dosing typically established?
   A I
   B II
   C III
   D IV

7. Which anatomical position is marked by the grey line?
   A Anterior border of the lash line
   B Anterior border of the orbicularis oculi
   C Anterior border of the tarsal conjunctiva
   D Anterior border of the tarsal plate

8. What is the predominant form of collagen in the matrix of the sclera?
   A Type I
   B Type II
   C Type V
   D Type VI

9. Which of the following is the most likely corneal endothelial cell density of a healthy 40-year-old human?
   A 500 cells/mm^2
   B 1,500 cells/mm^2
   C 2,500 cells/mm^2
   D 4,000 cells/mm^2

10. Which layer of the choroid lies furthest from the retina?
    A Bruch's membrane
    B Choriocapillaris
    C Haller's layer
    D Sattler's layer

11. What is the volume of the vitreous humour of an emmetropic adult?

    A 3 mL
    B 4 mL
    C 5 mL
    D 6 mL

12. Which of the following statements about skull osteology is true?

    A The coronal suture joins the frontal and temporal bones
    B The lambdoid suture lies above the pterion
    C The posterior fontanelle closes before the anterior fontanelle
    D The superciliary ridges are larger in females than males

13. Which one of the following statements about the Geneva lens measure is true?

    A It is calibrated for the refractive index of crown glass
    B It is possible to deduce the total power of a thin lens by measuring both surface powers and calculating the difference between them
    C It uses three spring-loaded pins to measure the surface curvature of a lens
    D When placed on a convex surface the central pin is extended relative to the peripheral pins

14. Which of the following statements about corneal innervation is false?

    A Fewer than 100 main stromal nerve bundles enter the cornea at the limbus
    B The inferior cornea is sometimes innervated by V2
    C The mid-stromal plexus is densest in the central cornea
    D Unmyelinated nerve fibres pierce Bowman's membrane to form the sub-basal plexus

15. What magnitude of accommodation will be required for a hypermetropic patient with a +2 dioptre prescription to read unaided at 20 cm?

    A 3 dioptres
    B 5 dioptres
    C 7 dioptres
    D 10 dioptres

16. Which of the following statements about the trabecular meshwork is false?

    A Contraction of the ciliary muscle reduces resistance to aqueous outflow across the trabecular meshwork
    B The cells of the juxtacanalicular meshwork are surrounded by an extracellular matrix
    C The corneoscleral meshwork has a lamellar structure
    D The uveal meshwork provides the greatest degree of resistance to aqueous humour outflow

17. Which of the following best describes the principal component of the lens zonules?

    A   Fibrillin
    B   Glycerol
    C   Lens epithelial cells
    D   Type IV collagen

18. Which of the following most accurately describes conjunctival microscopic anatomy?

    A   Most of the lymphoid tissue is located in the conjunctival epithelium
    B   The epithelium is stratified squamous in the palpebral and limbal portions
    C   The stroma in the palpebral conjunctiva is attached to Tenon's capsule
    D   Type V collagen is the main constituent of the epithelial basement membrane

19. Which of the following is not a typical route of toxoplasma infection?

    A   Contaminated drinking water
    B   Dog faeces
    C   Transplacental
    D   Undercooked meat

20. A 60-year-old man waiting for his diabetic eye clinic appointment develops chest pain. The electrocardiogram (ECG) shows ST elevation in leads V1–V4. Which coronary artery is likely to be blocked?

    A   Circumflex artery
    B   Left anterior descending artery
    C   Right coronary artery
    D   Right marginal artery

21. Regarding the optic nerve, which of these statements is incorrect?

    A   Axons arise from the retinal ganglion cells and synapse in the lateral geniculate body
    B   Myelin sheaths are formed from oligodendrocytes rather than Schwann cells
    C   There are approximately 3.7 million axons in the optic nerve
    D   The total length of the optic nerve is 4–5 cm

22. Regarding the primary visual cortex, which of the following is incorrect?

    A   Layer IV receives the optic radiations
    B   Layers V and VI project to the secondary visual cortex
    C   Macular function is represented posteriorly
    D   The contralateral upper visual field is represented below the calcarine sulcus

23. Which of the following are found in higher concentrations in the lens than in aqueous?

    A Glucose and potassium
    B Potassium and amino acids
    C Sodium and chloride
    D Water and glutathione

24. Which one of the following biochemical changes in the lens is not associated with cataract formation?

    A Increased glutathione levels
    B Increase in insoluble lens components
    C Loss of αA crystallin and γS crystallin
    D Protein cross-linking and aggregation

25. Regarding noradrenaline (norepinephrine), which of the following statements is false?

    A It is a hormone
    B It is a neurotransmitter
    C It is metabolised by monoamine oxidase
    D It is synthesised by catechol-O-methyltransferase

26. What is the degree of image magnification when viewing the fundus of a patient with 10 dioptres of myopia with a direct ophthalmoscope?

    A × 12.5
    B × 15
    C × 17.5
    D × 20

27. Which of the following best describes the lens epithelium?

    A A simple cuboidal epithelium covering the anterior lens surface
    B A simple cuboidal epithelium covering the posterior lens surface
    C A stratified cuboidal epithelium covering the anterior lens surface
    D A stratified cuboidal epithelium covering the posterior lens surface

28. Which of the following statements about retinal glucose metabolism is true?

    A 50% of glucose utilisation in the retina is by the photoreceptors
    B A high rate of aerobic respiration and a low rate of lactic acid production is characteristic
    C Glucose uptake in the retina is independent of insulin levels
    D The retina has a higher rate of aerobic glucose consumption than any tissue other than the liver

29. Which of the following best describes the basis of the dark current?
    A   An influx of potassium ions maintains a relative depolarisation of the photoreceptor
    B   An influx of potassium ions maintains a relative hyperpolarisation of the photoreceptor
    C   An influx of sodium ions maintains a relative depolarisation of the photoreceptor
    D   An influx of sodium ions maintains a relative hyperpolarisation of the photoreceptor

30. Which of these contributes to the blood–aqueous barrier?
    A   Capillaries in the ciliary processes
    B   Desmosomes in the pigmented ciliary epithelium
    C   Fenestrations in the iris capillaries
    D   Tight junctions in non-pigmented ciliary epithelium

31. Regarding the synthesis of melanin, select the incorrect statement.
    A   Deficiency of tyrosinase leads to albinism
    B   Melanin and adrenaline are derived from the same amino acid
    C   Melanin can be synthesised from phenylalanine
    D   Melanocytes are unable to produce melanin in vitiligo

32. Apoptosis can be triggered by internal or external factors. Which of these is not a trigger for programmed cell death?
    A   BAX
    B   BCL-2
    C   Fas ligand
    D   TNF-α

33. What is the approximate rate of cerebrospinal fluid production?
    A   50 mL/day
    B   150 mL/day
    C   300 mL/day
    D   550 mL/day

34. Which of the following is not an ocular effect of ionising radiation?
    A   Ablation of the retinal pigment epithelium and outer retina
    B   Cicatricial conjunctivitis
    C   Dry eyes
    D   Radiation retinopathy

35. Which one of the following bones of the orbit does not derive purely from membranous ossification?

    A   Lacrimal bone
    B   Maxilla
    C   Sphenoid
    D   Zygomatic bone

36. Which nerve in the cavernous sinus does not run along the lateral wall?

    A   Abducens nerve
    B   Maxillary nerve
    C   Oculomotor nerve
    D   Trochlear nerve

37. Regarding postnatal visual development, which of the following is typically present at birth?

    A   Accommodation
    B   Conjugate fixation reflex
    C   Primary fixation reflex
    D   Smooth pursuit

38. Which of the following hamartomatous conditions is not autosomal dominant?

    A   Neurofibromatosis type 1
    B   Sturge–Weber syndrome
    C   Tuberous sclerosis
    D   Von Hippel–Lindau syndrome

39. Which of the following techniques is used to study DNA?

    A   Eastern blot
    B   Northern blot
    C   Southern blot
    D   Western blot

40. During which stage of the cell cycle is DNA synthesised?

    A G_1
    B G_2
    C   M
    D   S

41. Which of these organisms is not normally part of the conjunctival or eyelid commensal flora?

    A   Coagulase-negative staphylococci
    B   Diphtheroids, e.g. *Corynebacteria*

C *Neisseria gonorrhoeae*
D *Streptococcus viridans*

42. Which one of the following genes is found on chromosome 13?

   A FBN1
   B PAX6
   C Rb
   D RP2

43. During cataract surgery on a patient with an eye of axial length of 23 mm, it becomes necessary to change intraocular lens type. The A constant for the original lens implant is 118.4, predicting a lens power of 21.5 dioptres. The A constant for the new lens is 117.4. What is the appropriate power for the new lens?

   A 20.5 dioptres
   B 21.0 dioptres
   C 22.0 dioptres
   D 22.5 dioptres

44. Which of the following statements about Robertsonian translocations is false?

   A Individuals with a balanced Robertsonian translocation are phenotypically normal
   B The prevalence of Robertsonian translocations is around 1 in 100,000
   C The vast majority of individuals with Robertsonian translocations have 45 chromosomes
   D Robertsonian translocations only occur in acrocentric chromosomes

45. Which of these does not contribute to normal retinal attachment?

   A Active transport of subretinal fluid by the retinal pigment epithelium (RPE)
   B Interdigitations of the photoreceptor outer segments and RPE microvilli
   C Proteins of the interphotoreceptor matrix
   D Tight junctions between RPE cells and the choriocapillaris

46. What is the time taken for migration of a photoreceptor disc from the base to the tip of the rod outer segment?

   A 10 minutes
   B 10 hours
   C 10 days
   D 10 weeks

47. After activation of a naïve T cell by an antigen presenting cell, which cytokine induces the clonal proliferation of the T cell?

    A IL-1
    B IL-2
    C IL-6
    D IL-8

48. Which of the following is not a major histocompatibility complex (MHC) class 1 antigen?

    A HLA-A29
    B HLA-B27
    C HLA-C
    D HLA-DR4

49. Which Purkinje-Sanson image is used in keratometry readings?

    A Image I
    B Image II
    C Image III
    D Image IV

50. Which of the following tests does not assess colour vision?

    A Farnsworth-Munsell
    B Hardy-Rand-Rittler
    C Ishihara
    D Pelli-Robson

51. Which of the following is not associated with HLA-B27?

    A Inflammatory bowel disease
    B Rheumatoid arthritis
    C Psoriatic arthritis
    D Uveitis

52. Which of the following stains is used to detect *Mycobacterium* species?

    A Giemsa
    B Hansel
    C Periodic acid–Schiff
    D Ziehl–Neelsen

53. Which of the following statements about endotoxins and exotoxins is true?

    A Endotoxins are lipopolysaccharides
    B Endotoxins are predominantly derived from Gram positive bacteria

C Exotoxins are constituents of the outer membrane of the bacterial cell wall
D Exotoxins are relatively heat-stable

54. Regarding the glands of the eyelids, which of the following statements is false?
    A The glands of Moll are modified sweat glands
    B The glands of Zeis are sweat glands
    C The glands of Zeis open into the eyelash follicles
    D The Meibomian glands are modified sebaceous glands

55. Which of the following statements about HIV is false?
    A High levels of p24 antigen are seen during the period between infection and seroconversion
    B HIV reverse transcriptase acts to create a DNA copy of virion RNA
    C HIV-1 was the first HIV subtype to be identified and is largely restricted to Africa
    D Langerhans cells are susceptible to HIV infection

56. Which of the following stains can be used for the rapid identification of fungi?
    A Calcofluor–white
    B Malachite–green
    C Masson's trichrome
    D Toluidine–blue

57. Which of the following is a bacterial virulence factor that results in the conversion of plasminogen to plasmin?
    A Coagulase
    B Hyaluronidase
    C Kallikrein
    D Streptokinase

58. In which plane are the deposits in macular drusen located in age-related macular degeneration?
    A Between Bruch's membrane and the retinal pigment epithelium (RPE)
    B Between the choriocapillaris and Bruch's membrane
    C Between the photoreceptor layer and the external limiting membrane
    D Between the RPE and the photoreceptor layer

59. Which of the following best describes the anatomy of Müller's muscle?
    A Arising from the anterior surface of the levator muscle, inserting into the skin of the superior palpebral sulcus
    B Arising from the anterior surface of the levator muscle, inserting into the superior border of the tarsus

C Arising from the underside of the levator muscle, inserting into the skin of the superior palpebral sulcus

D Arising from the underside of the levator muscle, inserting into the superior border of the tarsus

60. Which of the following statements about amphotericin is incorrect?

   A It binds ergosterol in cell membranes
   B It is ineffective against bacteria
   C It is ineffective against yeasts
   D It is known to cause fever and renal toxicity

61. A single nucleotide deletion in a gene will most likely result in which of the following?

   A Frame shift mutation
   B Missense mutation
   C Nonsense mutation
   D Silent mutation

62. Which of the following instruments relies on total internal reflection?

   A Direct ophthalmoscope
   B Fibre-optic intraocular illumination system
   C Gonioscopy lens
   D Operating microscope

63. Which of the following does not contribute to the relative immune privilege of the eye?

   A Corneal neovascularisation
   B Immunomodulatory molecules in the aqueous
   C The blood–ocular barrier
   D The spleen

64. Which of the following is a correct transcription of a 0.50 dioptre Jackson's cross-cylinder?

   A +0.25 DS/−0.25 DC
   B +0.25 DS/−0.50 DC
   C +0.50 DS/−0.25 DC
   D +0.50 DS/−0.50 DC

65. Which of the following statements about the iris is false?

   A The collarette lies at the pupil margin and marks the end of the posterior iris epithelium
   B The dilator pupillae muscle is derived from the anterior iris epithelium

C The dilator pupillae muscle lies deep to the iris stroma and has a radial arrangement

D The sphincter pupillae muscle has a concentric arrangement

66. Connexins are characteristic of which type of intercellular junctions?

A Desmosomes
B Gap junctions
C Tight junctions
D Zonulae adherentes

67. A patient is fitted with a rigid gas permeable contact lens. Their average K reading is 7.67 mm, and the base curve of the contact lens is 7.5 mm. What is the shape of the resultant tear lens?

A Concave
B Convex
C No tear lens will be formed
D Plano

68. Which of the following statements about basal cell carcinomas is false?

A Over 90% of malignant eyelid tumours are basal cell carcinomas
B Patients with Gorlin–Goltz syndrome are likely to develop basal cell carcinomas at a young age
C Sclerosing basal cell carcinomas may spread below normal epidermis
D Untreated basal cell carcinomas commonly metastasise to the liver

69. In a myopic patient, which of the following is increased with contact lens wear compared to glasses?

A Aniseikonia
B Image distortion
C Image magnification
D Optical aberrations

70. Which of the following prisms causes inversion of the image, without deviation or lateral transposition?

A Dove prism
B Fresnel prism
C Porro prism
D Wollaston prism

71. Which of the following structures is not an extension of Tenon's capsule?

A The fascial sleeve of the superior oblique muscle
B The levator aponeurosis

C The medial check ligament
D The suspensory ligament of Lockwood

72. Which of the following describes the image formed by a thin concave lens?
   A Real, erect, magnified, further from lens than object
   B Real, inverted, magnified, outside the second focal point
   C Virtual, erect, diminished, inside the second focal point
   D Virtual, inverted, diminished, at infinity

73. What is the inheritance pattern of Gorlin–Goltz syndrome?
   A Autosomal dominant
   B Autosomal recessive
   C X-linked dominant
   D X-linked recessive

74. Which of the following lasers causes its principal effect through photodisruption?
   A Argon laser
   B Cyclodiode laser
   C Excimer laser
   D Nd:YAG laser

75. What name is given to the superior transverse suspensory ligament of the upper eyelid?
   A Berry's ligament
   B Lockwood's ligament
   C Whitnall's ligament
   D Wieger's ligament

76. Which of the following best describes the fluid content of the cornea and the sclera?
   A Cornea: 50% hydrated. Sclera: 60% hydrated
   B Cornea: 60% hydrated. Sclera: 50% hydrated
   C Cornea: 70% hydrated. Sclera: 80% hydrated
   D Cornea: 80% hydrated. Sclera: 70% hydrated

77. A patient's prescription is +4.00 DS/−2.50 DC axis 90°. What is the toric transposition of this to the base curve +6 D?

   A $\dfrac{-4.50 \text{ DS}}{+6.00 \text{ DC axis } 90°/+8.50 \text{ DC axis } 180°}$

   B $\dfrac{-4.00 \text{ DS}}{+8.50 \text{ DC axis } 180°/-2.50 \text{ DC axis } 90°}$

C $\dfrac{+1.50 \text{ DS}}{+6.50 \text{ DC axis } 90°/+2.50 \text{ DC axis } 180°}$

D $\dfrac{+4.00 \text{ DS}}{-6.00 \text{ DC axis } 90°/+3.50 \text{ DC axis } 180°}$

78. A Maddox rod is placed in front of a patient's right eye with its axis vertical. She is asked to look at a white spotlight and sees a horizontal red line with the light above it. What does this indicate?

    A Esophoria
    B Exophoria
    C Right hyperphoria
    D Right hypophoria

79. Which of the following lenses can be used to examine the anterior chamber angle?

    A 90 dioptre lens
    B Hruby lens
    C Three mirror lens
    D Widefield lens

80. Which of the following statements about mydriasis is false?

    A There is an increase in spherical aberration
    B There is an increase in the influence of the Stiles–Crawford effect
    C There is an increased depth of field
    D There is decreased diffraction of light

81. Which of the following indirect ophthalmoscopy lenses gives the greatest magnification?

    A 15 D
    B 20 D
    C 28 D
    D 30 D

82. Regarding the facial bones, which of the following statements is true?

    A The maxillary sinus opens into the nose above the middle concha
    B The nasal cavity is split by the bony nasal septum, which is principally formed by the nasal bone
    C The nasolacrimal canal is formed by the nasal and lacrimal bones, and by the inferior nasal concha
    D The vomer and the mandible are the only unpaired facial bones

83. How far does the uniocular visual field extend horizontally?
    A 90°
    B 120°
    C 150°
    D 180°

84. Which of the following statements about the Galilean telescope is false?
    A It has an extremely narrow field of view
    B It is composed of two convex lenses
    C The image is typically dimmer than seen with the unaided eye
    D The objective and eyepiece lenses are separated by the difference between their focal lengths

85. Which MacCallan stage of trachoma is characterised by contraction of the palpebral conjunctival stroma?
    A Stage I
    B Stage II
    C Stage III
    D Stage IV

86. Langhans cells in granulomas are formed from the fusion of which inflammatory cells?
    A Basophils
    B Lymphocytes
    C Macrophages
    D Neutrophils

87. Which of the following statements about acute retinal necrosis is true?
    A It is characterised by necrotising retinitis in the absence of vitritis
    B The majority of cases are triggered by bacterial infection
    C There is a discrete border around the foci of retinal necrosis
    D There is a higher incidence in immunocompromised patients

88. What is the prismatic effect (in prism dioptres) of a 4 dioptre lens that has been decentred by 30 mm?
    A 0.75
    B 12
    C 30
    D 120

89. Regarding herpes zoster (varicella zoster virus) infections, which of the following statements is true?

    A   Aciclovir prevents entry of the virus into the host cell
    B   Cranial nerve involvement occurs in 80% of shingles cases
    C   They are caused by an RNA virus
    D   Uveitis is often associated with raised intraocular pressure

90. Graves' disease and myasthenia gravis are manifestations of which type of hypersensitivity reaction?

    A   Type I
    B   Type III
    C   Type IV
    D   Type V

91. Which of the following best reflects the mechanism of action of quinolones?

    A   Inhibition of folate synthesis
    B   Inhibition of protein synthesis
    C   Interference with DNA replication
    D   Lysis of bacterial cell walls

92. Regarding calcification, which of the following statements is false?

    A   Band keratopathy is associated with chronic uveitis
    B   Band keratopathy is associated with subepithelial calcium deposition
    C   Calcium is usually deposited in tissue as hydroxyapatite crystals
    D   Chronic renal failure may give rise to dystrophic calcification of the eye

93. Which of these is not typically associated with chronic inflammatory reactions?

    A   Amyloid deposition
    B   Giant cells
    C   Necrosis
    D   Neutrophil activation

94. Which one of the following is not derived from the hyaloid artery?

    A   Bergmeister's papilla
    B   Central retinal artery
    C   Förster-Fuchs' spot
    D   Mittendorf's dot

95. Which of the following is a selective antagonist at the β_1 adrenoceptor?

    A   Apraclonidine
    B   Betaxolol

C Levobunolol
D Timolol

96. Which of the following is an effect of carbonic anhydrase inhibition?

    A An increase in intraocular pressure
    B Catalysis of the hydration of carbon dioxide to carbonic acid
    C Hyperkalaemia
    D Metabolic acidosis

97. A 25-year-old woman is referred to the eye clinic with a large left pupil. There is a poor reaction to light on the left, but a slow, exaggerated near response with slow redilatation. Which pharmacological agent could be used to confirm the likely diagnosis?

    A Cocaine 4%
    B Hydroxyamphetamine 1%
    C Phenylephrine 2.5%
    D Pilocarpine 0.1%

98. Which of the following statements most accurately describes the action of corticosteroids?

    A They act on membrane-bound G-protein-coupled receptors
    B They affect gene transcription
    C They have an immediate pronounced anti-inflammatory action
    D They increase the production of prostanoids

99. Which of the following statements regarding anaesthetic drugs is false?

    A Glycopyrrolate and atropine can be used to blunt the oculocardiac reflex
    B Inhalational anaesthetic agents are associated with a rise in intraocular pressure
    C Intraocular pressure is reduced by all intravenous anaesthetic induction agents apart from ketamine
    D Suxamethonium causes a rise in intraocular pressure

100. What is the most common site of metastasis from a choroidal melanoma?

    A Bone
    B Liver
    C Lung
    D Skin

101. Which of the following statements regarding heparin is false?

    A Low-molecular-weight heparins potentiate the inactivation of factor Xa by antithrombin, but have limited effect on thrombin
    B Heparin may cause paradoxical thrombosis, due to thrombocytosis

C Protamine is a strongly basic protein which reverses the effects of unfractionated heparin

D Side effects of unfractionated heparin include hyperkalaemia and osteoporosis

102. Which of the following mydriatics has the longest duration of action?

A Atropine 1%
B Cyclopentolate 1%
C Homatropine 2%
D Tropicamide 1%

103. Which of the following medications has serious haematological side effects?

A Chloramphenicol
B Fusidic acid
C Latanoprost
D Sodium cromoglycate

104. Which of the following statements regarding aciclovir is true?

A It inhibits the DNA polymerase of the host cell
B It is a thymidine derivative
C Its effects are highly specific to herpes simplex and cytomegalovirus
D It requires phosphorylation to become active

105. Which one of the following conditions is not caused by triplet repeat expansion?

A Huntington's disease
B Myotonic dystrophy
C Spinocerebellar ataxia
D Tay-Sachs disease

106. The mass electrical response of the retina when stimulated by a bright flash of light is tested using which of the following electrophysiological techniques?

A Electrooculogram
B Full-field electroretinogram
C Multifocal electroretinogram
D Visual-evoked potential

107. Regarding cardiac function and Starling's law of the heart, which of the following statements is correct?

A Amyloidosis may cause cardiac failure by reducing afterload
B An increase in contractility increases end-systolic volume
C Aortic stenosis results in reduced stroke volume
D Starling's law states that the rate of myocardial contraction is proportional to muscle fibre length

108. Regarding haemoglobin:
    A Adult haemoglobin (HbA) contains two α polypeptide chains and two γ chains
    B Haem contains iron in the ferrous (Fe^{3+}) state
    C Thalassaemia results in the production of abnormal globin chains
    D The oxygen binding affinity of haemoglobin is reduced by acidity

109. Which of the following statements regarding the retinal pigment epithelium (RPE) is true?
    A Bruch's membrane is responsible for maintaining the blood–retinal barrier
    B Each RPE cell interdigitates with a single photoreceptor cell
    C Melanin granules and phagosomes are abundant in the cytoplasm
    D The RPE is responsible for opsin synthesis

110. What is the normal average rate of aqueous humour production?
    A 2.5 μL/min
    B 5.0 μL/min
    C 7.5 μL/min
    D 10.0 μL/min

111. Which of the following best describes the image produced by a triangular prism?
    A Erect, virtual, displaced towards the apex
    B Erect, virtual, displaced towards the base
    C Inverted, virtual, displaced towards the apex
    D Inverted, virtual, displaced towards the base

112. Which layers of the right lateral geniculate nucleus receive inputs from the right eye?
    A 1, 3 and 5
    B 1, 4 and 6
    C 2, 3 and 5
    D 2, 4 and 6

113. Which cranial nerve innervates the fourth pharyngeal arch?
    A Facial nerve
    B Glossopharyngeal nerve
    C Trigeminal nerve
    D Vagus nerve

114. In compound myopic astigmatism:
    A Both focal lines are behind the retina
    B Both focal lines are in front of the retina

C   One focal line is on the retina while the other is in front
D   The focal lines are straddling the retina

115. What percentage of the ocular circulation passes through the uveal tract?
    A   28%
    B   48%
    C   78%
    D   98%

116. Which of the following optic nerve targets is thought to deal with the afferent arm of the pupillary light reflex?
    A   Parvocellular reticular formation
    B   Pretectal nucleus
    C   Pulvinar nucleus
    D   Suprachiasmatic nucleus

117. Which of the following is not a recognised function of intrinsically photosensitive retinal ganglion cells?
    A   Auditory/visual integration
    B   Modulating circadian rhythm
    C   Pupillary light reflex
    D   Regulating the sleep cycle

118. Regarding gene therapy, which of the following is a disadvantage of using viral vectors?
    A   They are inefficient at transducing DNA
    B   They are not generally good at targeting a specific group of cells
    C   They can only carry a limited amount of genetic material
    D   They tend to replicate and thus destroy cells

119. The central corneal thickness is measured in 100 eyes and the standard deviation is calculated to be 25 μm. What would be the standard error of the mean?
    A   0.0025 μm
    B   0.025 μm
    C   0.25 μm
    D   2.5 μm

120. Which one of the following structures is not transmitted through the foramen ovale?
    A   Accessory meningeal artery
    B   Emissary veins
    C   Greater petrosal nerve
    D   Mandibular division of the trigeminal nerve

Questions: CRQs

12 CRQs to be answered in 2 hours

1. An 82-year-old woman presents with two painless nodular skin lesions, one on each lower lid. They were pointed out to her several months ago. Following assessment both lesions are excised. Histopathology slides are shown below.

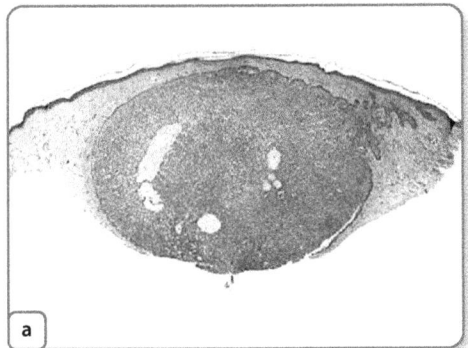
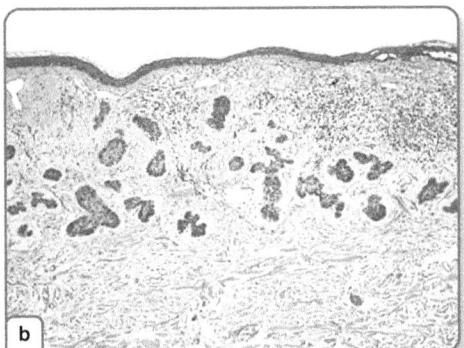

The pathology report confirms basal cell carcinoma (BCC).

(a) From which layer of the cutis does this tumour arise? (1 mark)
(b) Of the two slides above, which is the more concerning subtype and why? (2 marks)
(c) What is the principal form of spread? (1 mark)
(d) What further information do you require from the pathologist? (1 mark)
(e) Give two non-genetic risk factors for this type of skin cancer. (2 marks)
(f) Which clinical subtype of BCC is most likely to be successfully treated with topical imiquimod? (1 mark)
(g) Name two genetic conditions associated with early onset of multiple BCCs. (2 marks)

2.

(a) A +10.0 dioptre lens at a back vertex distance of 12 mm corrects a patient's refractive error. What power of lens will be required if the back vertex distance is changed to 7 mm? Please show your working. (2 marks)
(b) Draw two ray diagrams to demonstrate the change in the refractive effect of a convex lens as it is moved away from the eye. (4 marks)
(c) What form of image distortion may be encountered with a +10.0 lens in a spectacle prescription? (1 mark)
(d) The +10.0 lens in the right side of a pair of glasses is displaced 2 mm temporally. What will be the resultant prismatic effect for this eye? (1 mark)

(e) The prismatic effect of high-powered convex lenses increases towards the periphery. What symptoms do patients experience because of this? (2 marks)

3. A 29-year-old woman presents with a 2 months history of increasingly prominent eyes, pain which is worse on eye movements, intermittent redness, and watering. She has diplopia when looking to the right. She is a smoker and mentions that her periods recently stopped. Her GP performed blood tests last week which showed free thyroxine (T_4) of 30 and undetectable thyroid stimulating hormone (TSH).

(a) Which thyroid autoantibody is most likely to be positive? (1 mark)
(b) Give four systemic clinical signs that may be associated with this condition. (4 marks)
(c) Why might it be useful to obtain a urine sample from this patient? (1 mark)
(d) Given her symptoms, name two other hospital-based health professionals who should be involved in this patient's care. (2 marks)
(e) Give two sight-threatening complications of this condition. (2 marks)

4.

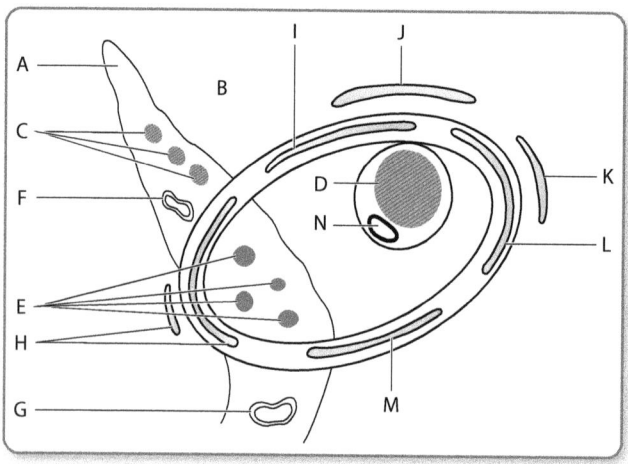

(a) Identify the fissure labelled A and the bone labelled B. (1 mark)
(b) Identify the nerves labelled C (in any order) and the nerve labelled D. (2 marks)
(c) Identify the nerves labelled E (in any order). (2 marks)
(d) Identify the structures labelled F and G. (1 mark)
(e) Indicate the motor nerve supply for each of the muscles labelled H–M. (3 marks)
(f) Indicate the clinical consequences of acute occlusion of the blood vessel labelled N. (1 mark)

5. A 58-year-old woman complains of unilateral blurred vision for the past 2 months. Visual acuity in the affected eye is 6/18 with a near vision of N14. Imaging is performed (**Figures a** and **b**).

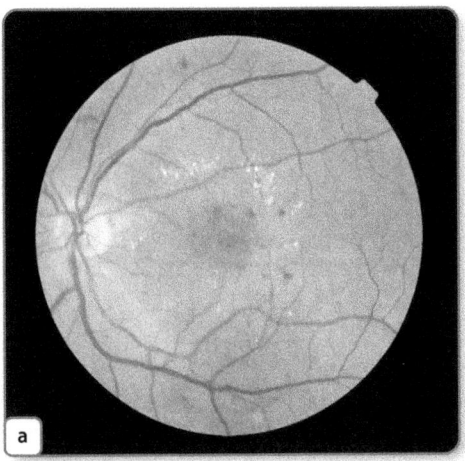
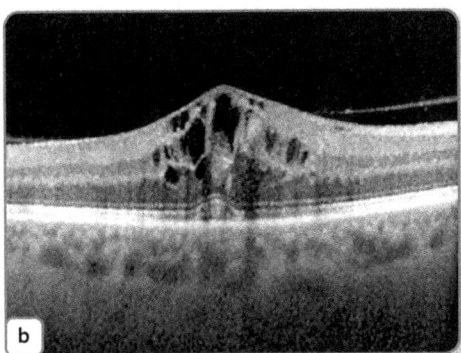

(a) State two abnormalities on the fundus photo. (2 marks)
(b) What is the name of the investigation shown in **Figure b**? (1 mark)
(c) Considering both the clinical presentation and investigations, what is the most likely diagnosis? (1 mark)
(d) Name two standard first-line treatments for this condition and briefly state the mode of action. (4 marks)
(e) Disregarding the fundus photo (**Figure a**), please name two other conditions which could cause the appearances seen in **Figure b**. (2 marks)

6. A 73-year-old woman with a background of type 2 diabetes mellitus presents to the emergency eye clinic with a sudden onset of painless horizontal binocular diplopia. A Hess screen is performed:

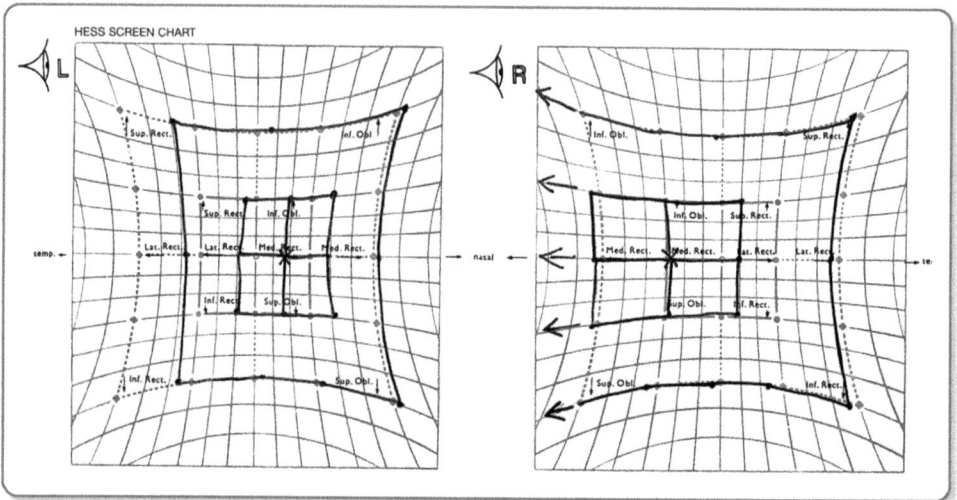

(a) Pathology of which cranial nerve is suggested by the Hess screen? (2 marks)
(b) Give three possible aetiologies for this cranial nerve disorder. (3 marks)
(c) State the anatomical location of the nucleus of this cranial nerve. (1 mark)
(d) Orthoptic examination reveals an esotropia for distance measuring 30 prism dioptres. Which Fresnel prism(s) could be fitted to the patient's distance glasses to control the diplopia? Give two options. (2 marks)
(e) Draw a ray diagram showing the refraction of light by a Fresnel prism. (2 marks)

7.
  (a) The figure below is a diagram of an embryo at 27 days. Name the structures labelled A–D. (4 marks)

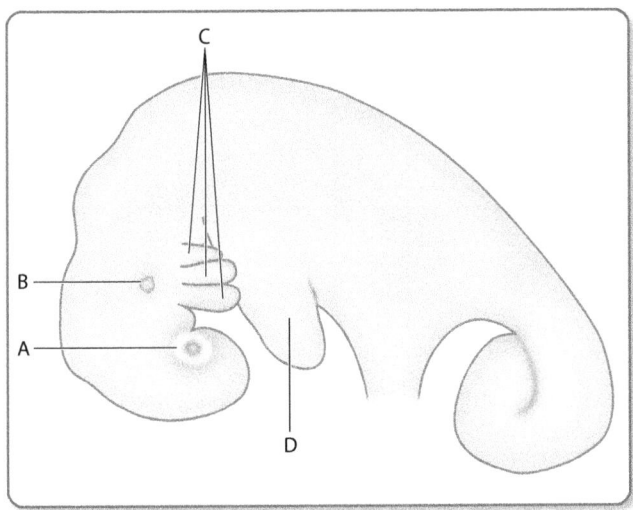

  (b) The figure below is a diagram of the developing eye at 27 days. Name the structures labelled A–D (4 marks)

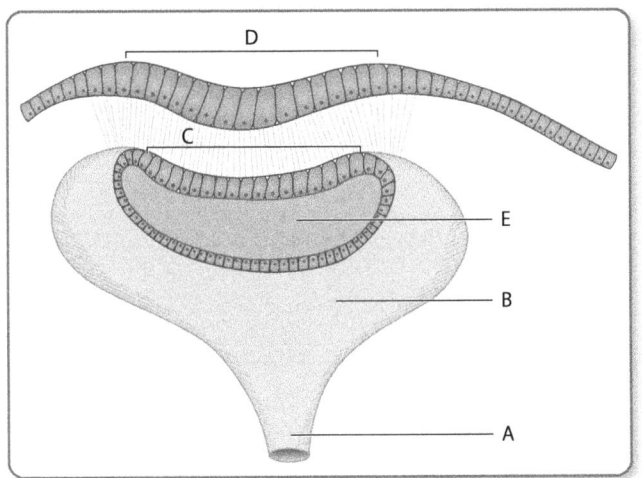

  (c) Which space will the cavity labelled E become? (1 mark)
  (d) After how many weeks does the lens vesicle separate from the surface ectoderm? (1 mark)

8.
   (a) Which optical aberration is illustrated by this image? (1 mark)

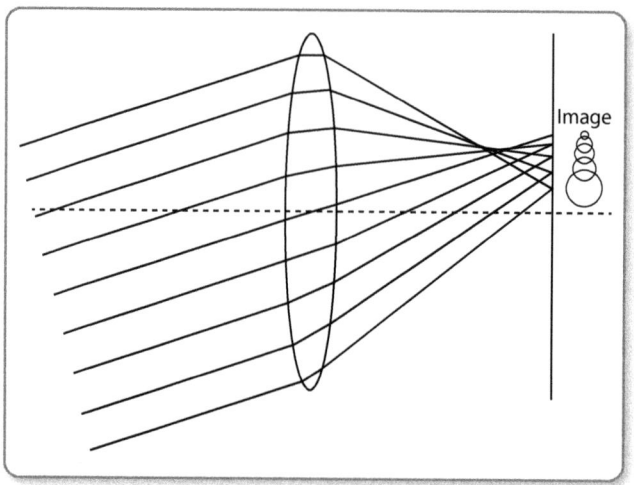

   (b) Which pathological condition is this aberration commonly seen in? (1 mark)
   (c) Which optical aberration is utilised in the duochrome test? (1 mark)
   (d) Draw a ray diagram illustrating the duochrome test. Clearly label the focal points of red and green light, and the retinal positions in low hypermetropia, emmetropia and low myopia. (5 marks)
   (e) How would you modify the duochrome test if you were testing a patient who was red-green colour blind? (1 mark)
   (f) Which optical aberration is principally responsible for the reduction in visual acuity following instillation of tropicamide eye drops? (1 mark)

9. This 70-year-old patient has a history of laser photocoagulation several years ago.

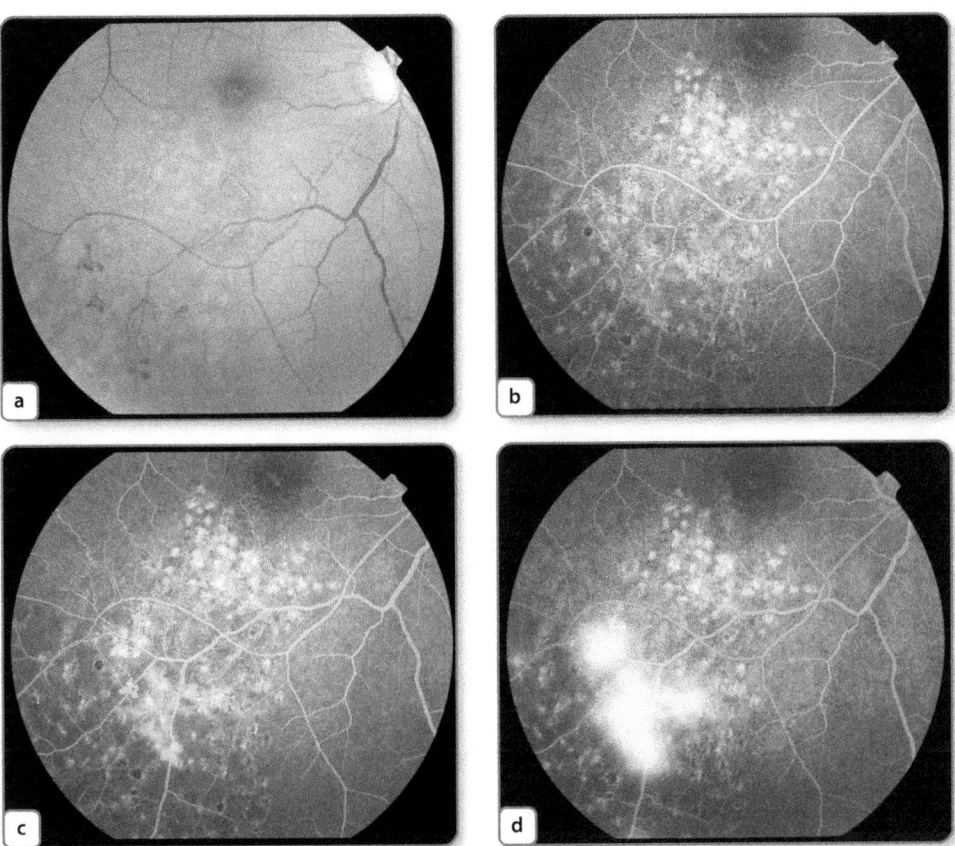

(a) Describe the two main vascular abnormalities on the red–free fundus image (**Figure a**). (2 marks)
(b) What are the most likely causes of the two types of abnormal hyperfluorescence on this fluorescein angiogram (**Figures b** to **d**)? (2 marks)
(c) Given that the areas of the fundus not imaged above are entirely normal, what is the likely aetiology of these findings? (1 mark)
(d) Explain briefly the 2 principles underlying fundus fluorescein angiography. (2 marks)
(e) What is the most serious potential side effect of fluorescein administration? (1 mark)
(f) Please give two common side effects of fluorescein. (2 marks)

10. A 3-day-old baby develops purulent discharge and lid swelling (**Figure a**). A conjunctival swab is taken and the organism identified stains pink/red on a Gram stain. An electron micrograph of the organism is shown in **Figure b**.

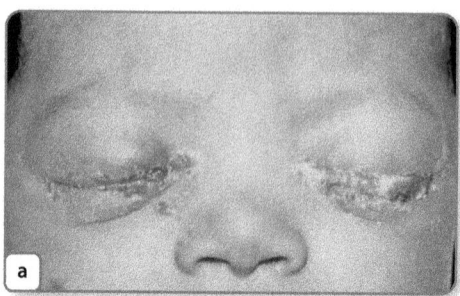
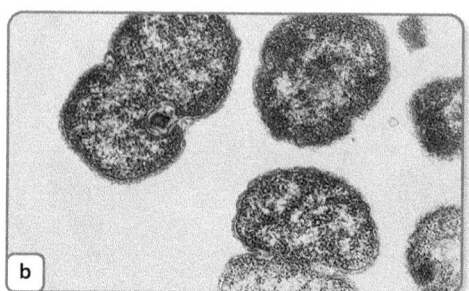

   (a) What is the diagnosis? (1 mark)
   (b) Which organism is most probably responsible? (1 mark)
   (c) Name a culture medium that can be used to grow this organism. (1 mark)
   (d) How is the infection acquired in neonates? (1 mark)
   (e) Give two sight-threatening complications which can occur as a result of corneal ulceration in this condition. (2 marks)
   (f) Is topical or systemic antimicrobial therapy more appropriate? (1 mark)
   (g) Name another organism that commonly causes this condition, and give two tests that can be performed to identify this organism. (3 marks)

11. Please answer the following questions regarding the compound microscope.

   (a) Draw a labelled ray diagram to explain how an image is produced by a compound microscope. (4 marks)
   (b) Briefly state the similarities and differences between the compound microscope and the astronomical telescope. (2 marks)
   (c) In a compound microscope intended for clinical use, what could be incorporated to usefully alter the nature of the image produced? Please draw a ray diagram illustrating the component you propose to add. (3 marks)
   (d) Explain how a slit lamp uses compound microscopes to give a binocular, stereoscopic view. (1 mark)

12. A study is investigating a new medication to reduce the recurrence of wet age-related macular degeneration (AMD) in patients who have previously been treated with anti-vascular endothelial growth factor (VEGF) injections. The recruited patients are randomised to receive either the new medication (intervention group) or a placebo (control group). Neither the patients nor the investigators are aware of which group each patient is in during the course of the study. The patients were followed up for a 2-year period.

The recurrence rate in the placebo group was 30% and the recurrence rate in the treatment group was 20%.

(a) What type of study design is this? (2 marks)
(b) The mean age of the patients in the intervention arm was 78 and the median age was 82. Explain how these values are calculated. (2 marks)
(c) What is the relative risk reduction? (1 mark)
(d) What is the number needed to treat for this intervention? (1 mark)
(e) What is the null hypothesis in this study? (1 mark)
(f) Describe a type I error, both in general terms and relating to this study. (2 marks)
(g) The study concludes that there is a difference between the recurrence rates in the two groups with a P value of 0.04 (Student's t-test). What does this tell you about the probability of the observed difference being due to chance? (1 mark)

Answers: SBAs

1. **B Neural crest mesenchyme**

   The lens vesicle (an invagination of surface ectoderm) separates in week 5. The surface ectoderm reconnects anteriorly to the forming lens, and will become the corneal epithelium. Neural crest-derived mesenchymal cells then migrate in waves into the space that will later become the anterior chamber. The trabecular meshwork, corneal endothelium, corneal stroma and the iris stroma all arise from these cells.

2. **B Between the centre of curvature and the principal focus**

   A real, inverted and enlarged image from a concave mirror arises when an object is between the centre of curvature and the principal focus. It is always worth drawing the ray diagram for these questions. One ray runs from the top of the object parallel to the principal axis, and is reflected through the principal focus. The other runs from the top of the object through the centre of curvature and will therefore hit the mirror at 90° to the surface, and be reflected along the same path. The image is formed where these two rays intersect (see Figure 1.1, page 50). Note that because the question gives information on where the image lies it is possible to draw the diagram in reverse, starting with the image and tracing back through the centre of curvature and principal focus.

3. **D Vancomycin**

   Vancomycin (a glycopeptide antibiotic) is ineffective against Gram negative bacteria as it cannot penetrate their outer membrane. Cefuroxime is a second generation cephalosporin and has broad coverage of both Gram positive and Gram negative bacteria. Amoxicillin is an aminopenicillin and has activity against some Gram negative (in addition to multiple Gram positive) organisms. Metronidazole, a nitroimidazole, is active against most Gram negative and Gram positive anaerobes as well as many protozoans.

4. **B Dichroic**

   Polarised light consists of light waves which are all orientated in the same plane. Polarisation can be achieved by different methods, such as selective absorption (e.g. in dichroism), reflection, scattering or the use of birefringent materials. Polarisation results in a reduction in intensity, but spectral composition is unaffected.

   The property described in the question is dichroism. A dichroic substance only allows the transmission of light in an incident plane aligned with its structure by absorbing light waves in other planes.

   There are naturally occurring crystalline dichroic substances, and manufactured ones, the best known being polaroid. Polaroid was originally composed of iodoquinine crystals embedded in plastic, although several variants have been developed.

5. **C 6.9 mm**

The origin of the four rectus muscles is the common tendinous ring or annulus of Zinn. Their insertions onto the sclera are measured in millimetres posterior to the limbus (**Table 3.1**). The closest to the limbus is the medial rectus, followed by inferior, lateral and then superior rectus. The medial rectus has the shortest tendon; the lateral rectus has the longest. The lateral rectus has a small second head arising from the orbital surface of the greater wing of sphenoid (lateral to the annulus of Zinn).

Table 3.1 Insertions of rectus muscles	
Muscle	Insertion (mm from limbus)
Medial rectus	5.5
Inferior rectus	6.5
Lateral rectus	6.9
Superior rectus	7.7

6. **B II**

The different phases of clinical trials are outlined in **Table 3.2**. These are the phases of studies in humans and do not encompass all the previous laboratory and animal testing that a potential drug undergoes before entering clinical trials. Note that phase 0 trials and phase IV trials do not always occur.

Table 3.2 Phases of clinical trials		
Clinical trial phase	Principal aim	Subjects
0	Human microdosing studies to establish safety	Healthy volunteers or target group of patients; usually <20 subjects
I	Assess principally safety and side effects, but also tolerability, pharmacokinetics and pharmacodynamics	Healthy volunteers or target group of patients; usually <100
II	Phase IIA: establish dosing Phase IIB: establish efficacy	Target group of patients; usually <300
III	Determine effectiveness, in particular effectiveness versus current gold standard; usually randomised clinical trials	Target group of patients; typically 1,000–3,000
IV	Postmarketing surveillance to detect side effects; further studies to continue to assess effectiveness (e.g. in different populations)	Target group; thousands of patients

7. **D Anterior border of the tarsal plate**

   The grey line is a key landmark for a number of surgical procedures involving the eyelid and corresponds histologically to a superficial portion of the pretarsal orbicularis oculi (known as the muscle of Riolan), which marks the anterior border of the tarsal plate. The skin/conjunctival transition zone lies posterior to this, at the level of the Meibomian gland openings.

8. **A Type I**

   The matrix of the sclera is predominantly composed of type I collagen. A number of other collagen types have been detected in the sclera in smaller quantities (including types III, IV, V, VI, VIII, XII and XIII). Interestingly the corneal stroma is also principally composed of type I collagen, but the laminar construction is highly regular, as opposed to the sclera which has an irregular arrangement of collagen and elastic fibres.

9. **C 2,500 cells/mm^2**

   Corneal endothelial cell density in a healthy adult is normally approximately 2,500 cells/mm^2. 3,000–4,000 cells/mm^2 may be seen in a child's cornea, and in old age this usually falls to around 2,000 cells/mm^2. Pathological conditions, such as Fuchs' endothelial dystrophy, and iatrogenic causes, such as cataract surgery, may lower the endothelial cell count further and can lead to corneal decompensation.

10. **C Haller's layer**

    The choroid is usually described in terms of four layers, listed below (**Table 3.3**) from the outermost (and therefore furthest from the retina) to the innermost. Some sources include the suprachoroid in this list: this transition zone lies outside Haller's layer.

    Table 3.3 Layers of the choroid

Layer	Features
Haller's layer	Larger calibre arteries and veins
Sattler's layer	Intermediate calibre arterioles and venules
Choriocapillaris	Dense bed of fenestrated capillaries Only extends to the ora serrata anteriorly
Bruch's membrane	Acellular connective tissue layer Further subdivided into 5 layers (see page 36, question 15)

11. **B 4 mL**

    The vitreous humour of an emmetropic adult is approximately 4 mL and therefore the vitreous accounts for approximately two-thirds of the total volume of the eye. The vitreous is approximately 99% water and therefore its mass in grams is approximately equal to its volume in mL.

12. C The posterior fontanelle closes before the anterior fontanelle

The posterior fontanelle is the first to close and usually closes 2–3 months after birth, whereas the anterior fontanelle closes last of all fontanelles at between 12 and 36 months.

The coronal suture joins the frontal and parietal bones. The lambdoid suture is the posterior suture joining the occipital and parietal bones. Its anterior ends form part of the asterion.

The superciliary ridges are larger in males than females (in some females they are absent altogether). This difference develops through puberty.

13. A It is calibrated for the refractive index of crown glass

The Geneva lens measure is calibrated for crown glass and gives a direct reading in dioptres. The power of lenses of other materials may be calculated if the refractive index is known. The total power of a thin lens is equal to the sum of both surface powers. There are three pins on a Geneva lens measure, but only the central pin is spring-loaded. The peripheral pins are fixed, and the reading is based on the position of the mobile central pin relative to the fixed peripheral pins. When placed on a convex surface the central pin is retracted relative to the peripheral pins (it is extended when placed on a concave surface).

14. C The mid-stromal plexus is densest in the central cornea

The cornea is principally innervated by nerves from V1 via the long ciliary nerves. In a small number of individuals there is some innervation of the inferior cornea from branches of V2.

Some 50–90 main stromal nerve fibres enter the cornea at the limbus in a radial direction. Perineurium and myelin sheaths are lost from these nerves near the limbus to preserve corneal clarity. They travel in the anterior half of the stroma, branching to form a mid-stromal nerve plexus. This is densest in the peripheral cornea and decreases in both density and complexity towards the central cornea.

Most mid-stromal nerve fibres pass anteriorly within the stroma and form a subepithelial plexus below Bowman's membrane. Nerves arising from this plexus pierce Bowman's membrane to pass anteriorly and form a plexus below the basal aspect of the corneal epithelium. From this sub-basal plexus, the sensory nerve endings arise to supply the corneal surface (there are more sensory nerve endings per unit area than anywhere else in the body).

15. C 7 dioptres

The accommodation required by an emmetropic patient to read unaided at a given distance is equal to the reciprocal of the distance in metres. In this case therefore the accommodative power required for an emmetropic patient would be 1/0.2, i.e. 5 dioptres. However, a patient with a +2 dioptre prescription will require 2 dioptres of accommodation to see an object clearly at infinity and therefore the total accommodation required to focus at 20 cm will be 7 dioptres.

For this reason the onset of presbyopia is earlier in hypermetropic patients than in emmetropic patients (the onset in low myopic patients is even later). See page 141, feedback to question 75, for an alternative method for approaching this type of problem.

16. **D The uveal meshwork provides the greatest degree of resistance to aqueous humour outflow**

    The uveal meshwork is the first layer of the trabecular meshwork that the aqueous must pass through and has large intercellular spaces, and consequently a low resistance to aqueous flow. The next layer is the corneoscleral meshwork, which is a lamellar structure of connective tissue covered by endothelium-like cells. The final layer is the juxtacanalicular or 'cribriform' meshwork, which is embedded in an extracellular matrix composed of collagen, elastic fibres and proteoglycans. Contraction of the ciliary muscle causes expansion of the three-dimensional structure of the trabecular meshwork which results in enlargement of the intertrabecular spaces, and therefore reduction of the resistance to aqueous outflow.

17. **A Fibrillin**

    The lens zonules are composed of microfibrils that are principally non-collagenous. The major constituent is fibrillin, a glycoprotein. They share similar properties to elastin, giving both tensile strength and elasticity. The fibrillar elements are surrounded by a layer of glycosaminoglycans (including hyaluronate) and other glycoproteins. This coating may include type IV collagen. Lens zonules are acellular.

18. **B The epithelium is stratified squamous in the palpebral and limbal portions**

    The conjunctiva is a translucent mucous membrane composed microscopically of three layers (**Table 3.4**).

Table 3.4 Properties of the layers of the conjunctiva	
Conjunctival epithelium	Non-keratinised, 2–7 layers: • Stratified squamous (palpebral and limbal) • Stratified columnar (bulbar) Other cells: goblet cells, melanocytes, dendritic cells, lymphocytes
Conjunctival epithelial basement membrane	Type IV collagen Anchoring fibrils and hemidesmosomes
Conjunctival stroma	Loose connective tissue: • Superficial lymphoid layer • Deep collagenous fibrous layer attached to Tenon's/episclera (apart from palpebral conjunctiva, where it adheres to tarsal plate)

Answers: SBAs

19. **B Dog faeces**

    The *Toxoplasma gondii* parasite reproduces in the intestinal mucosa of the cat, which is the definitive host, and the cysts pass into cat faeces. Other animals can ingest cysts from contaminated soil and become intermediate hosts, but dog faeces are more commonly a source of *Toxocara canis* infection.

    Human infection is acquired following ingestion of cysts, either from contact with cat faeces, from contaminated and undercooked meat, or contaminated drinking water. Transplacental infection can also occur resulting in congenital toxoplasmosis.

20. **B Left anterior descending artery**

    ST changes in leads V1–V4 suggest an anteroseptal infarct. This region is supplied by the left anterior descending artery.

    The right coronary artery supplies the inferior (leads II, III and aVF) and posterior (reciprocal changes in leads V1–V3) areas. The right marginal artery is a branch of the right coronary artery.

    The circumflex artery supplies the lateral area (leads I, aVL and V5–V6).

21. **C There are approximately 3.7 million axons in the optic nerve**

    The optic nerve runs from the disc to the chiasm and is approximately 4–5 cm long. It is comprised of intraocular (1 mm), orbital (2.5 cm), intracanalicular (0.5–1 cm) and intracranial (1–1.5 cm) portions. Beyond the chiasm, the nerve fibres continue as the optic tracts.

    It is composed of approximately 1.2 million axons, which arise from the retinal ganglion cells and synapse in the lateral geniculate body. Interestingly, during foetal development, optic nerve axons peak in number at around 16 weeks' gestation (3.7 million) and then decline to adult levels by the 3rd trimester.

    The optic nerve is myelinated posterior to the optic disc, with the myelin coming from oligodendrocytes (as it does in the central nervous system) rather than Schwann cells.

22. **B Layers V and VI project to the secondary visual cortex**

    The primary visual cortex is also known as V1, the striate cortex or Brodmann's area 17. It occupies the area around the calcarine sulcus on the medial surface of each occipital lobe. There is a sophisticated topographic representation of the retina within V1. Each primary visual cortex represents the contralateral visual field, with the upper field being represented below the calcarine sulcus and vice versa. The peripheral retina is represented anteriorly and the macula posteriorly. There are six layers in the primary visual cortex (**Table 3.5**).

Table 3.5 Layers of the primary visual cortex	
Layer(s)	Connections
I	Predominantly composed of dendritic and axonal connections
II III	Project to secondary visual cortex
IV	Receives optic radiations from the lateral geniculate nucleus
IV V	Project to superior colliculus
VI	Projects to lateral geniculate nucleus

23. **B Potassium and amino acids**

    Table 3.6 compares the biochemical composition of aqueous and the lens, and outlines the principal modes of exchange of these substances. In addition to the table below, ascorbic acid is found in a higher concentration in the lens than in aqueous.

    The lens behaves chemically (and electrically) somewhat like a single cell, with barriers to transport and active pumping mechanisms occurring particularly at the capsule and epithelial cell membranes. Gap junctions within the lens also contribute to this.

Table 3.6 Biochemical composition of the aqueous and the lens			
	Aqueous	Mode of exchange	Lens
Water	99%	Osmosis	66%
Amino acids	5 mmol/L	Active transport	25 mmol/L
K^+	5 mmol/L	Active transport	120 mmol/L
Na^+	144 mmol/L	Active transport	10–20 mmol/L
Cl^-	110 mmol/L	Diffusion	18 mmol/L
Glucose	6 mmol/L	Diffusion	1 mmol/L
Glutathione	0 mmol/L	(Synthesised in the lens)	12 mmol/L

24. **A Increased glutathione levels**

    There are several biochemical changes in the lens associated with cataract formation, including:

    - Cross-linking (particularly disulphide bonds) and aggregation of lens proteins
    - Increased susceptibility to oxidative damage, including a reduction in glutathione levels
    - Loss of αA crystallin and γS crystallin

    These changes can result in reduced transparency and a change in both the colour (yellowing) and refractive index of the lens.

25. D It is synthesised by catechol-O-methyltransferase

Noradrenaline is a catecholamine that acts as both a neurotransmitter (in the sympathetic nervous system and hypothalamus) and a hormone (released by the adrenal medulla).

Structurally, it differs from adrenaline only by a methyl group. Both are tyrosine derivatives. The immediate precursor in the synthesis pathway is dopamine: the enzyme dopamine β-hydroxylase converts dopamine to noradrenaline. The further addition of a methyl group to the terminal amine gives adrenaline.

Monoamine oxidase (MAO) and catechol-O-methyltransferase (COMT) metabolise rather than synthesise noradrenaline. The action of noradrenaline as a neurotransmitter is terminated either by reuptake into the postganglionic nerve ending, or by degradation by COMT or MAO.

26. C × 17.5

When the fundus is viewed with a direct ophthalmoscope the eye acts as a simple magnifier, therefore the degree of magnification can be found using the formula:

$$M = \frac{F}{4}$$

Where M is the magnification and F is the refracting power in dioptres. From the schematic eye we know that the total refracting power of the emmetropic eye is approximately 60 dioptres.

Therefore, a patient with 10 dioptres of myopia will have a total refracting power of approximately 70 dioptres and the magnification will be:

$$\frac{70}{4} = 17.5 \times$$

There is a degree of simplification when using this approach. For example, in reality there is a difference in the magnification produced by refractive versus axial myopia. Nonetheless it is important to understand the basic principles of how magnification of a direct ophthalmoscope is calculated, and how it varies with ametropia.

27. A A simple cuboidal epithelium covering the anterior lens surface

The lens epithelium is a simple cuboidal epithelium (i.e. cuboidal cells in a single layer) and is restricted to the anterior lens surface. Near to the lens equator the cell morphology changes to be more columnar. The cells continue to elongate and become lens fibres.

28. C Glucose uptake in the retina is independent of insulin levels

The uptake of glucose in the retina is regulated by the extracellular concentration of glucose rather than by insulin. Photoreceptors have a retina-specific insulin receptor that has a steady state of activity independent of hyper- or hypoglycaemic states. The photoreceptors account for over 80% of glucose utilisation in the retina. There is a high rate of both aerobic and anaerobic respiration in the retina, with a high rate of lactic acid production. The rate of aerobic glucose consumption in the retina is higher than any other tissue in the body, including the liver.

29. C An influx of sodium ions maintains a relative depolarisation of the photoreceptor

The dark current depends on the influx of sodium ions into the photoreceptor through cyclic GMP-gated ion channels in the outer segment during conditions of darkness. As these ions are positively charged this induces a relative depolarisation of the photoreceptor to around −40 mV, compared with a resting membrane potential of around −70 mV in most neurons. The outer segments of photoreceptors lack Na^+/K^+ ATPase pumps, therefore, the sodium ions flow down a concentration gradient to the inner segment where Na^+/K^+ ATPase pumps are present and can extrude sodium ions from the cell.

30. D Tight junctions in non-pigmented ciliary epithelium

The blood-aqueous barrier is maintained by:

- Tight junctions between non-pigmented ciliary epithelial cells
- Iris capillaries, which are non-fenestrated and have tight junctions between vascular endothelial cells

The capillaries in the ciliary processes are fenestrated and therefore do not contribute to the barrier. Desmosomes are found between the internal surfaces of the pigmented ciliary epithelial cells but do not form part of the blood–aqueous barrier.

31. D Melanocytes are unable to produce melanin in vitiligo

Melanin is derived from the amino acid tyrosine, which can be synthesised from phenylalanine. A simplified synthetic pathway is shown in **Figure 3.1**.

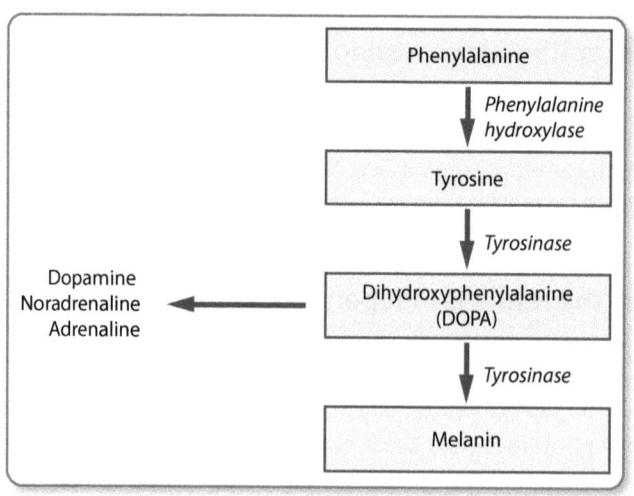

Figure 3.1 Synthesis of melanin.

In vitiligo lesions, melanocytes are absent. In albinism, they are present, but melanin production is impaired. Deficiency of the tyrosinase enzyme (which catalyses the rate-limiting step) is one mechanism by which this occurs.

32. **B BCL-2**

Programmed cell death is a tightly regulated process, with BCL-2 being an important inhibitor of apoptosis. Internal stress or damage to a cell causes activation of BAX, a protein from the same family as BCL-2, which activates apoptosis, principally via cytochrome C release from mitochondria. A number of other cellular proteins have since been identified as apoptosis modulators, and disruption of apoptosis-regulating proteins have been implicated in various cancers. External stimuli including Fas ligand and TNF-α also activate apoptosis through several mechanisms, including cascades activated by specific cell surface receptors.

33. **D 550 mL/day**

Cerebrospinal fluid (CSF) is produced at a rate of approximately 550 mL/day. Given that the total CSF volume is 125–150 mL this means the CSF turns over approximately four times a day. Production is from the choroid plexus and the ventricle walls, and reabsorption is principally via the arachnoid villi with a small contribution from the cerebral venules.

34. **A Ablation of the retinal pigment epithelium and outer retina**

The eye is affected by both ionising and non-ionising radiation. Ionising means that the radiation has enough quantum energy to eject an electron from an atom or molecule. Ablation of the retinal pigment epithelium and outer retina occurs in laser photocoagulation, which is non-ionising radiation.

Ionising radiation may be composed of particles moving at relativistic speeds (e.g. electrons, neutrons) or high energy electromagnetic radiation. The threshold for ionising lies within the ultraviolet range of the electromagnetic spectrum (**Figure 3.2**, see below).

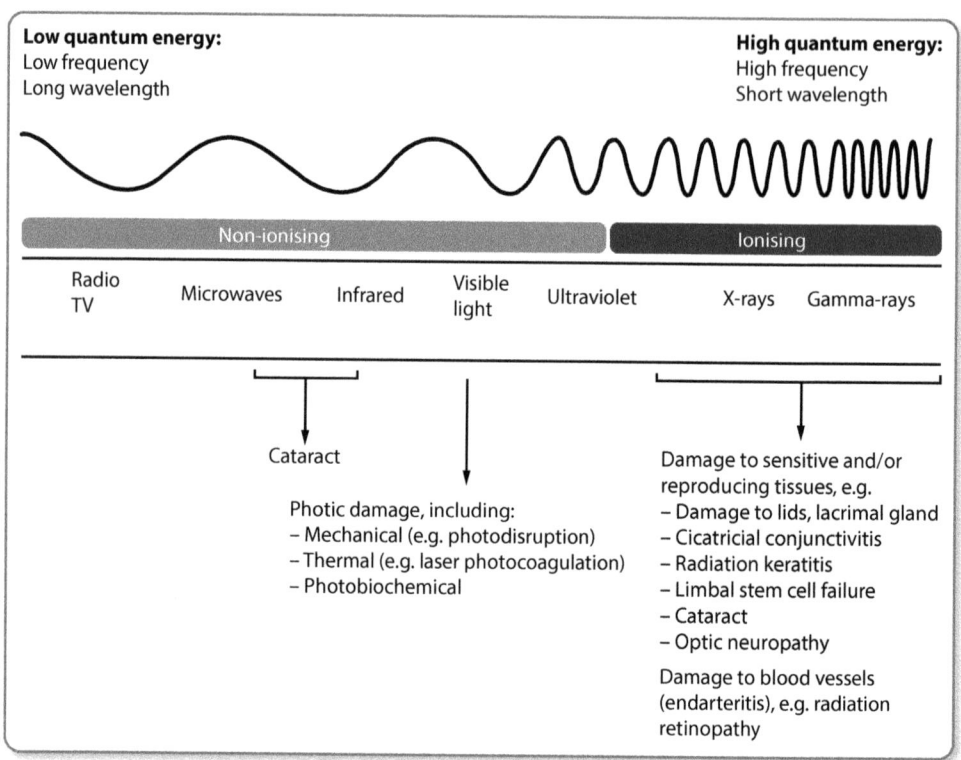

Figure 3.2 Ocular damage due to radiation.

35. C Sphenoid

The skull base initially forms as cartilaginous precursors which subsequently ossify to form the midline of the skull base. In the orbit the body, the lesser wing and the medial section of the greater wing of the sphenoid ossify in this way. Parts of the ethmoid bone also ossify from cartilage. The remainder of the bones of the orbit are derived from membranous ossification, i.e. they do not have a cartilaginous precursor.

36. A Abducens nerve

The abducens nerve runs freely within the cavernous sinus, whereas the other nerves run along the lateral wall: from superior to inferior these are the oculomotor nerve (III), trochlear nerve (IV), ophthalmic nerve (V1) and maxillary nerve (V2). See diagram in Paper 1, CRQ 1 on page 23 and 71.

37. C Primary fixation reflex

The primary fixation reflex, whereby fixation occurs with either eye, is typically present at or immediately after birth. The eye movements may be grossly conjugate and may diverge, but rarely converge.

The macula remains poorly developed at this stage. The fovea develops in the first few months of life, with increased cone density and myelination of the nerve fibres in the visual pathway.

The ability to move the eyes together to take up fixation during versions is called the conjugate fixation reflex, and develops from 2 to 3 weeks of age.

Smooth pursuit and accommodation develop from 2 months. Convergence develops by 6 months.

38. B Sturge–Weber syndrome

Sturge–Weber syndrome is the result of a somatic mosaic variant in the *GNAQ* gene. This genetic mutation occurs after fertilisation (it is not inherited). By contrast, neurofibromatosis type 1, tuberous sclerosis and Von Hippel–Lindau syndrome are inherited in an autosomal dominant fashion (although the mutations may arise *de novo*: if this happens then the mutation will subsequently be inherited in an autosomal dominant manner). The genes responsible are listed in **Table 3.7**.

Table 3.7 Selected genes associated with hamartomatous conditions		
Condition	Gene	Chromosome
Neurofibromatosis type 1	*NF-1*	17q
Tuberous sclerosis	*TSC1* and *TSC2*	9q and 16p
Von Hippel–Lindau syndrome	*VHL*	3p

39. C Southern blot

Southern blotting was invented by Edwin Southern and can be used to detect a particular sequence of DNA within a complex mixture. Subsequent blotting techniques have been developed, including the Northern blot to detect RNA, the Western blot to detect specific proteins, the Eastern blot to detect post-translational protein modifications, and the Southwestern blot to detect specific DNA-binding proteins.

40. D S

DNA is synthesised during S phase, which stands for synthesis phase. Each chromosome replicates. G_1 phase is a 'gap' phase which occurs prior to S phase. During G_1 the cell increases in size and synthesises required mRNA and proteins. Cells can remain in G_1 for days if required, before proceeding to S phase. Following S phase the cell enters the G_2 phase, where the cell synthesises further proteins and grows in preparation for mitosis. After G_2 the cell enters a mitotic 'M' phase, undergoing mitosis and cytokinesis.

41. C *Neisseria gonorrhoeae*

The normal commensal flora of the conjunctiva and eyelids helps to prevent pathogenic colonisation. The commonest commensals are typically coagulase-negative staphylococci, such as *Staphylococcus epidermidis*. Several other Gram positive organisms contribute to the normal flora, including aerobes, such as *Staphylococcus aureus*, *Micrococcus*, and *Corynebacteria*, and anaerobes, such as *Propionibacteria*.

Gram negative organisms are also identified as commensals, albeit less frequently. These include *Moraxella*, *Escherichia* and *Proteus* species.

By contrast, *Neisseria gonorrhoeae* is an important cause of serious neonatal conjunctivitis.

42. C Rb

Retinoblastoma is associated with mutations in both alleles of the *Rb* gene (sometimes referred to as *RB1*), which is a tumour suppressor gene found on the long arm of chromosome 13.

Marfan's syndrome is inherited in an autosomal dominant manner and is associated with *FBN1* gene mutations on chromosome 15, which encodes the protein fibrillin-1. Mutations of the *PAX6* gene on chromosome 11 are associated with a range of disorders of ocular development.

Retinitis pigmentosa (RP) describes a collection of different rod–cone dystrophies and so has a variety of inheritance patterns. Genes associated with RP include the *RP2* and *RPGR* genes, associated with X-linked RP, and the *RHO* (rhodopsin) gene on chromosome 3 (autosomal dominant RP).

43. A 20.5 dioptres

The SRK formula can be reasonably applied to eyes of normal axial length:

$$P = A - B(AL) - C(K)$$

Where P is the required IOL power; A is a constant that is dependent on the model of lens used; B is a constant (calculated as 2.5); C is a constant (calculated as 0.9); AL is the measured axial length of the eye and K is the average keratometry.

As the formula is a summation with no modifying variable to the A constant, a change in the A constant will directly correspond to a change in the required IOL power.

In this case the difference is:

$$117.4 - 118.4 = -1$$

Therefore, the lens power for the new lens type will also be 1 dioptre less, i.e. 20.5 dioptres.

44. B The prevalence of Robertsonian translocations is around 1 in 100,000

The prevalence of Robertsonian translocations is around 1 in 1,000, and it is therefore one of the most common forms of chromosome rearrangements in humans.

In Robertsonian translocations, the long arms of two acrocentric chromosomes fuse to form a single chromosome. The short arms of acrocentric chromosomes generally contain non-essential genetic material and are quickly lost following a Robertsonian translocation. This leaves the individual with an essentially complete set of genetic data and a resultant normal phenotype, but typically only 45 chromosomes. There is a subsequent increased risk of trisomy in offspring, dependent on the chromosomes involved and compatibility with life (**Figure 3.3**). Monosomy is not compatible with life.

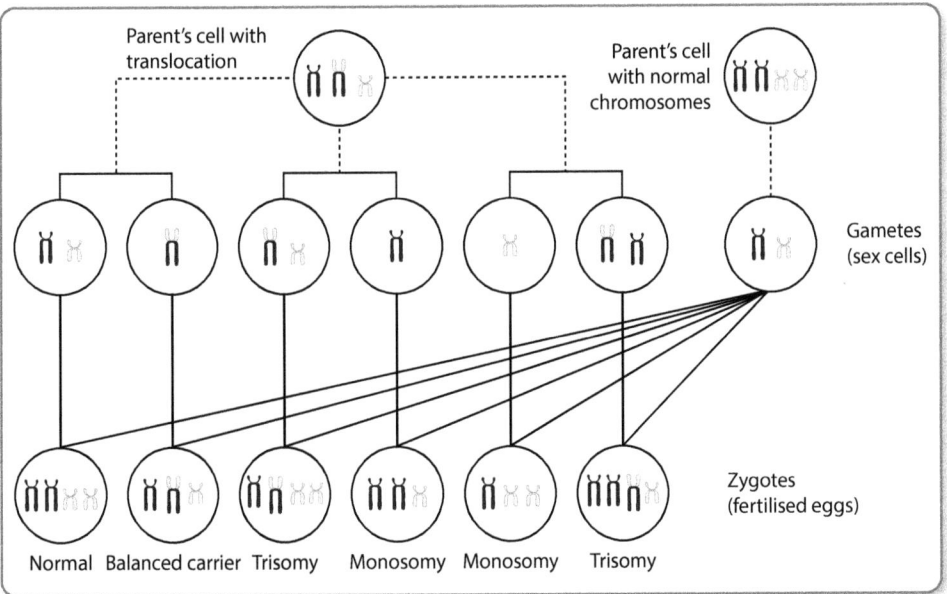

Figure 3.3 Roberstonian translocation.

45. **D Tight junctions between RPE cells and the choriocapillaris**

Adhesion of the neurosensory retina to the retinal pigment epithelium (RPE) is maintained under normal circumstances by several physiological forces. Structurally, there are interdigitations between the outer segments of the photoreceptors and the RPE microvilli. Proteins and glycosaminoglycans of the interphotoreceptor matrix (between the retina and RPE) promote retinal attachment.

The blood–retinal barrier is sustained by tight junctions between endothelial cells of retinal vessels and between RPE cells. There are no tight junctions between RPE cells and the choriocapillaris.

Fluid dynamics are crucial in keeping the retina transparent and apposed to the choroid. The net direction of passage of fluid from the vitreous through the retina is outward. This is due to active pumping of fluid by RPE cells, as well as the relative oncotic pressures of the vitreous and choroid.

46. **C 10 days**

Photoreceptors are highly metabolically active and undergo constant turnover. Renewal of photoreceptors occurs by new membrane synthesis at the outer limiting membrane along with shedding of the tips of the outer segment. Discs form at the junction between the inner and outer segments, and, in rod photoreceptors, it takes 10 days for migration of a disc to the tip of the outer segment. This is therefore the time it takes for complete renewal of the outer segment. Discs are shed in a diurnal pattern and phagocytosed by the retinal pigment epithelium.

47. **B IL-2**

Interleukins are so called because of their important role in inter-leucocyte communication. Following activation by an antigen presenting cell, T cells develop interleukin-2 (IL-2) receptors and start to produce IL-2. IL-2 acts in an autocrine fashion to induce the clonal proliferation of that T cell.

IL-2 is thus the principal cytokine involved in T cell clonal proliferation. Elevated levels of IL-2 are found in patients with active eye inflammation, for example uveitis.

48. **D HLA-DR4**

Human leucocyte antigen (HLA)-A, -B and -C are examples of major histocompatibility complex (MHC) class 1 antigens. The presence of particular MHC antigens can be relevant clinically in ophthalmology. For example, HLA-A29 is associated with a form of posterior uveitis called birdshot chorioretinopathy, and individuals with an HLA-B51 allele have a higher relative risk of Behçet's disease. The HLA-D molecules, for example HLA-DR4, are MHC class 2 antigens.

49. **A Image I**

Purkinje–Sanson images are formed from the reflection of light at the air–cornea interface (image I), the cornea–aqueous interface (image II), the aqueous–lens interface (image III) and the lens–vitreous interface (image IV). Images I, II and III are erect virtual images (convex reflecting surfaces), whereas image IV is an inverted real image (concave reflecting surface). Image I is used in keratometry to assess the anterior corneal surface.

50. **D Pelli–Robson**

The Pelli–Robson chart is used to assess contrast sensitivity. Farnsworth–Munsell 100 hue testing requires the subject to arrange four rows of similarly coloured tiles in the appropriate order. Hardy–Rand–Rittler and Ishihara tests are both based on pseudoisochromatic plates. Ishihara plates test for protan and deutan deficits (red–green colour blindness), while Hardy–Rand–Rittler plates additionally test for tritan deficits.

Answers: SBAs

51. B Rheumatoid arthritis

Human leucocyte antigen-B27 (HLA-B27) is associated with:

- Uveitis (commonly recurrent, unilateral anterior uveitis)
- Seronegative spondarthritides, e.g. ankylosing spondylitis, psoriatic arthropathy, reactive arthritis
- Inflammatory bowel disease

A significant proportion of uveitis cases are associated with HLA-B27. However, in straightforward cases, e.g. non-granulomatous, unilateral anterior uveitis that responds rapidly to treatment, with no systemic symptoms, the blood test for HLA-B27 is not always performed, as it does not alter treatment.

Blood testing for HLA-B27 is positive if one copy of the gene is present. HLA-B27 has a strong association with the above conditions, but is not a diagnostic test for them. It is not useful in asymptomatic individuals. The UK population prevalence of HLA-B27 is approximately 8% and many of this group will never develop any of the conditions above. Only 1% of those who do have HLA-B27 will develop uveitis.

52. D Ziehl–Neelsen

Ziehl–Neelsen staining is used to detect acid-fast bacilli, such as *Mycobacterium*. These species are resistant to traditional Gram staining techniques.

53. A Endotoxins are lipopolysaccharides

Endotoxins are lipopolysaccharides and are constituents of the outer membrane of the cell wall of Gram negative bacteria. They are relatively heat stable, as opposed to exotoxins which are easily damaged by heat. Exotoxins are proteins which are either secreted by living bacteria or released during cell lysis (endotoxins are almost exclusively released upon cell lysis). Endotoxins are exclusively derived from Gram negative bacteria whereas exotoxins may be produced by both Gram positive and Gram negative bacteria.

54. B The glands of Zeis are sweat glands

The thin skin of the eyelids is continuous with the conjunctiva at the lid margin and contains numerous glands as well as the lash follicles. The lash follicles, which do not have erector pili muscles, form two to three rows along the anterior border of the lids. The glands of Zeis are sebaceous glands which open into each lash follicle. The modified sweat glands of Moll open either directly onto the lid margin or into the lash follicles. A stye, sometimes referred to as an external hordeolum, is an acute infection of one of these two types of gland or of a lash follicle.

In contrast to the above structures, which lie in the anterior lamella of the eyelid, the Meibomian glands lie within the tarsus in the posterior lamella. They are modified sebaceous glands.

55. **C HIV-1 was the first HIV subtype to be identified and is largely restricted to Africa**

   Human immunodeficiency virus (HIV)-1 was the first HIV subtype to be identified and has since spread globally. HIV-2 is less prevalent and less pathogenic, and has largely been restricted to western Africa, although cases have been reported in a number of other countries.

   Langerhans cells are susceptible to HIV infection and are likely initial targets of infection following exposure of mucous membranes to the virus.

   HIV reverse transcriptase produces an antisense DNA copy of the virion's RNA and then subsequently acts as a DNA-dependent DNA polymerase to create a corresponding sense DNA strand. These form a double-stranded viral DNA, which is then integrated into the host genome by the activity of the enzyme integrase.

   p24 antigen is a viral protein derived from the virion core. It is present in relatively high levels during the initial viral replication following infection, but becomes undetectable as the immune system responds during seroconversion (there is a corresponding increase in anti-p24). p24 antigen may become detectable again in later stages of the disease as the CD4 count and anti-p24 decrease.

56. **A Calcofluor–white**

   Calcofluor–white can be used in the rapid identification of fungi in samples as it binds to chitin and cellulose in cell walls. When excited by high frequency light it fluoresces a bluish–white colour. It can also be used in the detection of some parasitic organisms.

57. **D Streptokinase**

   Many pathogenic organisms produce substances that facilitate their spread through host tissues. These are a type of virulence factor, and include enzymes which break down connective tissue and blood clots. Streptokinase is a thrombolytic agent produced by some species of *Streptococci*, which causes the conversion of plasminogen to plasmin, which in turn dissolves fibrin. Whilst kallikrein also activates plasminogen, it is an endogenous serine protease and is not produced by bacteria.

58. **A Between Bruch's membrane and the retinal pigment epithelium (RPE)**

   Macular drusen are characterised histologically by focal deposits of extracellular debris between Bruch's membrane and the RPE. There is immune cell proliferation within the deposits, and this may lead to neovascularisation and/or fibrous metaplasia.

59. D Arising from the underside of the levator muscle, inserting into the superior border of the tarsus

Müller's muscle is a smooth muscle innervated by the sympathetic nervous system. It arises from the underside of the levator palpebrae superioris in the region of the aponeurotic–muscular junction, travels inferiorly between the levator aponeurosis and the conjunctiva and inserts onto the superior border of the tarsus. The levator aponeurosis inserts onto the anterior surface of the superior tarsal plate, with some fibres said to attach to the skin forming the upper lid skin crease. Müller's muscle provides additional elevation (1–2 mm) of the upper lid during periods of high sympathetic tone.

60. C It is ineffective against yeasts

Amphotericin is an antifungal and antiprotozoal agent that has been used for decades with a very low incidence of resistance. It binds ergosterol in fungal cell membranes and increases membrane permeability as well as inducing oxidative damage. It is very effective against yeasts, but not bacteria as their cell membranes do not contain ergosterol.

Amphotericin is usually given intravenously or topically. It is nephrotoxic, and its large side effect profile includes fever and hypokalaemia.

61. A Frame shift mutation

Insertions or deletions of nucleotides in groups not divisible by 3 will typically result in a frame shift mutation, as DNA codons are read in triplets. Missense mutations occur when a point mutation changes a codon from one amino acid to another. Nonsense mutations are point mutations that create a premature stop codon, and therefore an incomplete and often non-functional protein product. Silent mutations have no phenotypical consequences, and are generally either mutations in non-coding regions, or mutations that result in a different codon for the same amino acid or for an amino acid with similar properties. Note that as there are 64 possible codons and only 20 amino acids (and 'stop' codons) there is a degree of redundancy with multiple codons translating to the same amino acids.

62. B Fibre-optic intraocular illumination system

Fibre-optic intraocular illumination systems rely on total internal reflection to transmit light from an external light source to the instrument tip without loss of intensity *en route*. Gonioscopy lenses overcome total internal reflection in the cornea thanks to their refractive index. Direct ophthalmoscopes and operating microscopes do not rely on total internal reflection.

63. A Corneal neovascularisation

Ocular immune privilege serves to protect the clear media of the eye from the disruptive effects of immune-mediated inflammation, while maintaining some ability to fight pathogens. It is the product of several factors, including the blood–ocular barrier, a relative paucity of lymphatics in the eye, soluble immunomodulatory molecules in the aqueous (e.g. cytokines, neuropeptides, growth factors), and specialised tolerance-promoting antigen presenting cells. The latter requires an intact eye–spleen axis, and alters the body's response to eye antigens.

A well-known demonstration of the immune privilege of the eye is corneal transplantation. Corneal transplants, which are not usually HLA-matched, show a high rate of acceptance with only topical steroid medication. This is in contrast to other solid organ transplants. Corneal neovascularisation, however, is a risk factor for graft rejection as it brings blood into contact with the allograft.

64. B +0.25 DS/−0.50 DC

Jackson's cross-cylinders are toric lenses constructed so that the cylinder is twice the power of the sphere and of the opposite sign. This gives the effect of an equal and opposite dioptric power either side of zero, allowing the systematic testing of both the axis and power of the required cylinder during subjective refraction. The equivalent prescription for the above cross cylinder in plus cylinder format would be −0.25 DS/+0.50 DC. The cross-cylinders are designated by the power of their cylinder, so a 1.00 dioptre cross-cylinder would have a prescription of −0.50 DS/+1.00 DC.

65. A The collarette lies at the pupil margin and marks the end of the posterior iris epithelium

The collarette lies around 2 mm from the pupil margin and separates the iris into a pupillary and a ciliary zone. The iris is the thickest at this point, which marks the remnant of the minor vascular circle of the pupillary membrane. The dilator pupillae has a radial arrangement and is derived from the anterior iris epithelium lying immediately deep to the iris stroma. The sphincter pupillae muscle has a concentric arrangement and lies in the pupillary zone. Deep to the anterior iris epithelium is the posterior iris pigment epithelium, which is heavily pigmented. Note that iris colour is determined by the melanin production of melanocytes in the iris stroma.

66. B Gap junctions

Connexins are a family of transmembrane proteins that are the constituent parts of connexons, which are hemichannels between the cytoplasm of two cells. They are found at gap junctions, and each cell will provide a connexon so that a complete channel is formed. This allows signalling molecules, such as Ca^{2+}, to pass between cells, allowing multiple cells to co-ordinate their response. See page 128, Table 2.5 for a summary of intercellular junctions.

67. B Convex

Rigid gas permeable contact lenses have a fixed base curve, and therefore a 'tear lens' usually forms between the lens and the cornea. The shape of the tear lens will depend on the difference between the base curve of the contact lens and the

K readings of the cornea. If these are the same, a plano tear lens will be formed. If the K reading (in mm) is greater (i.e. flatter) than the base curve, as in this case, a convex tear lens will be formed. If the K reading is shorter (i.e. steeper) than the base curve then a concave tear lens will be formed.

68. D Untreated basal cell carcinomas commonly metastasise to the liver

Basal cell carcinomas almost never metastasise, although they invade into surrounding tissues. They are the most common form of malignant eyelid tumour, accounting for over 90% of cases.

Gorlin–Goltz syndrome (also known as nevoid basal cell carcinoma syndrome) is an autosomal dominant condition with a number of features including a predisposition to basal cell carcinomas. These usually occur at a young age and often multiple carcinomas develop.

There is a spectrum of clinical subtypes within basal cell carcinomas. Sclerosing (morphoeic) basal cell carcinomas can invade the dermis and spread outwards through this layer below normal epidermis. This contrasts with the classic nodular subtype, which typically has well-defined clinical margins.

69. C Image magnification

Myopes have greater image magnification with contact lenses compared to glasses, as they sit closer to the eye. The opposite is true for hypermetropes.

Aniseikonia is reduced with contact lens wear compared to glasses. This makes contact lenses useful in, for example, the correction of unilateral aphakia.

Image distortion can be troublesome with high-powered spherical lenses: 'barrel' distortion with concave lenses and 'pin-cushion' distortion with convex lenses.

When looking through the periphery of a lens, optical aberrations and an induced prismatic effect occur. By contrast, contact lenses move with the eyes such that the line of vision remains near the optical centre of the lens.

70. A Dove prism

Dove prisms are used to invert an image, but cause no deviation or lateral transposition. They are essentially a truncated right-angle prism, in which rays of light undergo total internal reflection (once) before emerging on the opposite side. Prisms such as these are often used in ophthalmic instruments. Contrast the Dove prism with Porro, Wollaston and Fresnel prisms by studying the ray diagrams on page 138, Figure 2.1.

71. B The levator aponeurosis

The fascial sheath that surrounds the eyeball is known as Tenon's capsule or fascia bulbi. Anteriorly, it attaches approximately 1.5 mm posterior to the limbus. It forms a thin membrane under the conjunctiva, separated from the sclera by the episcleral space and loose connective tissue. Posteriorly, it is continuous with the meninges around the optic nerve.

Various structures pierce Tenon's capsule, including the ciliary nerves and vessels, vortex veins and the extraocular muscle tendons. Where the muscle tendons pass through, the Tenon's capsule is reflected back to form a fascial sleeve. The sleeves for the medial and lateral recti expand to form the medial and lateral check ligaments, respectively, which attach to the lacrimal and zygomatic bones. Inferiorly, the fascial sheath thickens and becomes the suspensory ligament of Lockwood.

72. **C Virtual, erect, diminished, inside the second focal point**

The image formed by a thin concave lens has the same characteristics regardless of the position of the object: it is virtual, erect, diminished and inside the second focal point. This is in contrast to convex lenses, in which there are three scenarios for image formation, depending on the position of the object. See page 51, Figure 1.2, for ray diagrams.

73. **A Autosomal dominant**

Gorlin–Goltz syndrome has an autosomal dominant pattern of inheritance. It is caused by mutations in the *PTCH1* gene on chromosome 9, which produces the protein 'patched-1'. Patched-1 interacts with sonic hedgehog during development, and acts to suppress cell growth and division. Gorlin–Goltz syndrome is characterised by early development of multiple basal cell carcinomas, often during adolescence or early adulthood. Affected individuals also often develop benign tumours of the jaw and have a higher baseline risk of developing other forms of tumour.

74. **D Nd: YAG laser**

The Nd: YAG laser uses photodisruption, which is largely a mechanical effect, to break tissues apart (for example, in posterior capsulotomies). This is extremely useful as tissues may be opened or separated without entering the eye surgically. Argon and cyclodiode lasers cause photocoagulation and the excimer laser causes photoablation.

75. **C Whitnall's ligament**

Whitnall's ligament is a condensation of fascial tissue running horizontally just below the superior orbital rim from the lacrimal gland fascia to the trochlea. The levator muscle alters direction at Whitnall's ligament from horizontal to vertical, and thus the ligament acts as a fulcrum for the levator. It also provides support for the soft tissues of the superior orbit, particularly the lacrimal gland.

76. **D Cornea: 80% hydrated. Sclera: 70% hydrated**

The cornea maintains a higher level of hydration relative to other ocular tissues such as the sclera. However, it is capable of further hydration due to the high concentration of glycosaminoglycans and the dehydrating actions of the corneal endothelial pump. The sclera by comparison has a quarter of the proteoglycan and glycosaminoglycan content of the cornea.

77. **A** $\dfrac{-4.50\ \text{DS}}{+6.00\ \text{DC axis } 90°/+8.50\ \text{DC axis } 180°}$

The steps of toric transposition are outlined on page 56, feedback to SBA 78 in exam paper 1.

The key to getting this calculation right is first doing a simple transposition of the original prescription, to make the cylinder the same sign as the base curve:

+4.00 DS/−2.50 DC axis 90°

becomes:

+1.50 DS/+2.50 DC axis 180°

and this is the prescription you work with for the remainder of the steps.

78. **C Right hyperphoria**

The Maddox rod has been placed with the axis vertically over this patient's eye, so this will test for vertical deviations. The red line seen by the patient is horizontal and is displaced in the opposite direction to the ocular deviation. As the patient has seen the red line below the light, this means the right eye is displaced upwards. This is therefore a right hyperphoria. For further explanation of the Maddox rod, see page 55, feedback to SBA 74 in exam paper 1.

79. **C Three mirror lens**

The three mirror lens contains a mirror that allows visualisation of the anterior chamber angle, and so can be used to perform gonioscopy. The other two mirrors show the mid-peripheral and peripheral fundus, whilst the centre of the lens shows the posterior pole. Like a gonioscopy lens, it is a contact lens which overcomes the total internal reflection within the cornea that would normally prevent the angle from being seen.

80. **C There is an increased depth of field**

Mydriasis causes a decrease in the depth of field and the depth of focus. The depth of field is the range of distance an object can be moved within while still maintaining acceptable clarity. The depth of focus is the range of distance within which the image of an object will remain acceptably sharp at the retina. The converse is true of miosis, which increases both the depth of field and depth of focus. This can be seen when viewing objects in bright light, when using a pinhole or when triggering accommodation.

Mydriasis causes a decrease in the diffraction of light, as diffraction is greater with smaller apertures. Spherical aberration increases to the fourth power of pupil diameter, and it is this that is responsible for the greatest part of the blurred vision associated with mydriasis. Chromatic aberration also increases.

The Stiles–Crawford effect is the observation that photoreceptors respond less to light entering through the periphery of the lens than through the centre, possibly due to the orientation of the components of the retina. Increased pupil size causes an increase in light passing through the peripheral lens and therefore an increase in the influence of the Stiles–Crawford effect.

81. **A 15 D**

In indirect ophthalmoscopy, the magnification increases with decreasing power of examination lens, while the field of view decreases. The 15 D lens is used for high magnification viewing of the posterior pole. For further details of how these lenses are used, please see page 56, feedback to SBA 79 in exam paper 1.

82. **D The vomer and the mandible are the only unpaired facial bones**

The bridge of the nose is formed by the nasal bones, whereas the bony component of the nasal septum, which bisects the nasal cavity, is principally formed by the vomer. Along with the mandible, the vomer is unpaired. The remainder of the facial bones (zygomatic, maxilla, nasal, lacrimal, inferior nasal conchae and palatine) are all paired.

The bony nasolacrimal canal, which houses the nasolacrimal duct, is formed by the maxilla (not the nasal bone), lacrimal bone and inferior nasal concha (inferior turbinate). The canal is directed posteriorly, inferiorly and laterally. The nasolacrimal duct runs from the lacrimal sac to the inferior meatus, which is the space below the inferior concha. By contrast, the maxillary sinus opens into the nose via the hiatus semilunaris into the middle meatus, which is the space below the middle concha.

83. **C 150°**

The normal visual field of an eye extends 90–100° temporally and 60° nasally, giving a horizontal field of 150–160°. Vertically, it extends 70–80° inferiorly and 50–60° superiorly. Even in the absence of pathology, the real extent of the field also depends on the stimulus and background conditions.

Visual acuity is maximal at the point of fixation and decreases steeply nasally, and gradually temporally. The blind spot is an absolute scotoma 10–20° temporal to fixation.

84. **B It is composed of two convex lenses**

The Galilean telescope is composed of a convex objective lens and a concave eyepiece lens (see diagram on page 171). It has an extremely narrow field of view and a limited depth of focus. These limit its usefulness as a low vision aid, particularly since those needing low vision aids often have unsteady hands.

The image is typically slightly dimmer than seen with the unaided eye due to absorption and reflection of light by the two lenses of the system, in addition to the effects of the exit pupil. The objective and eyepiece lenses are separated by the difference between their focal lengths, as opposed to the astronomical telescope where the two convex lenses are separated by the sum of their focal lengths.

85. D Stage IV

There are two main grading systems for classifying trachoma progression: the MacCallan classification (**Table 3.8**), and the WHO simplified grading system (**Table 3.9**). Both systems are outlined below:

Table 3.8 MacCallan classification system	
Stage	Features
I	• Conjunctival hyperaemia • Early lymphoid hyperplasia • Oedema of the conjunctival stroma with infiltrating polymorphs
II	• Mature follicles and/or papillae • Peripheral corneal fibrovascular pannus formation
III	• Fibrous tissue formation • Obvious scarring of palpebral conjunctiva
IV	• Contraction of the palpebral conjunctival stroma • Secondary entropion, trichiasis and corneal damage

Table 3.9 WHO simplified grading system	
Grade	Signs
Trachomatous inflammation, follicular (TF)	≥5 follicles of >0.5 mm on upper tarsal conjunctiva
Trachomatous inflammation, intense (TI)	Inflammatory thickening obscuring >50% of normal deep tarsal vessels
Trachomatous conjunctival scarring (TS)	Cicatrisation of tarsal conjunctiva with visible white bands
Trachomatous trichiasis (TT)	Trichiasis of at least one lash
Corneal opacity (CO)	Corneal opacification involving part of the pupil margin

Fibrosis of the lacrimal gland, associated ducts and the accessory structures of the conjunctiva leads to a reduced tear film which exacerbates the process.

86. C Macrophages

Langhans cells are multinucleate giant cells which are formed from the fusion of epithelioid macrophages within a granuloma. The nuclei classically form a horseshoe shape around the periphery of the cell. They should not be confused with Langerhans cells, which are dendritic cells found in the skin and mucosal tissues.

87. **C There is a discrete border around the foci of retinal necrosis**

    Acute retinal necrosis (ARN) is characterised by:

    - Single or multiple foci of retinal necrosis with discrete borders
    - Occlusive vasculopathy with arteriolar involvement
    - Progression of disease in the absence of antiviral treatment
    - Vitritis and anterior chamber inflammation

    There may more rarely be optic nerve involvement. Retinal detachment can be a later complication. The most commonly implicated pathogens are varicella zoster virus and herpes simplex viruses 1 and 2. Less commonly, cytomegalovirus and Epstein–Barr virus can be the cause.

    ARN characteristically occurs in immunocompetent individuals, although there is a related entity in immunocompromised patients called progressive outer retinal necrosis (PORN). While both are believed to result from herpes virus infection, PORN does not typically have the associated vitritis, vasculitis or papillitis of ARN.

88. **B 12**

    Spectacle lenses may have a prismatic effect, either from decentration of the lens or from an incorporated prism. The amount of prism power induced by decentration of a lens can be calculated as follows:

    $$P = F \times D$$

    Where P is the prism power (in prism dioptres); F is the power of the lens (in dioptres); D is the decentration (in cm; note the value in the question was expressed in mm).

89. **D Uveitis is often associated with raised intraocular pressure**

    Herpes zoster infections are caused by varicella zoster virus, a double-stranded DNA virus and a member of the herpes family. The primary infection is in the form of chicken pox and the most common site for reactivation (shingles) is the thoracolumbar area. However, cranial nerve involvement occurs in around 20% of patients, with the ophthalmic division of the trigeminal nerve being the second most common site after the thoracolumbar area. Ocular involvement may involve inflammation in almost any ocular structure, with keratitis and uveitis being typical. Herpetic uveitis is characteristically associated with elevated intraocular pressure.

    Aciclovir is effective against herpes viruses but the mechanism of action is inhibition of viral DNA synthesis.

90. **D Type V**

    Myasthenia gravis and Graves' disease are autoimmune conditions that are both examples of type V hypersensitivity reactions. Antibodies recognise and bind to host cell surface receptors. For example, in Graves' disease, antibodies bind to and activate the thyroid-stimulating hormone (TSH) receptor, resulting in overactivity of the thyroid gland.

Type V is not part of the original Gell and Coombs classification, and in fact type V hypersensitivity reactions are categorised by some as a subclass of type II. However, unlike antibody-mediated cytotoxic type II reactions, in type V reactions the host cell is not destroyed. Furthermore, in type II reactions the antibodies bind to antigens on the host cell, but not to specific receptors.

91. **C Interference with DNA replication**

    Quinolones interact with bacterial DNA gyrase and topoisomerase IV, enzymes essential for bacterial DNA replication.

    Quinolones are broad-spectrum antibiotics which are commonly used in ophthalmology. Ciprofloxacin is given orally (or sometimes intravenously) and reaches therapeutic intraocular concentrations. Ofloxacin, moxifloxacin and levofloxacin are used topically in the treatment of bacterial keratitis.

92. **D Chronic renal failure may give rise to dystrophic calcification of the eye**

    Calcification is referred to as metastatic when it occurs in normal tissues, classically in the presence of hypercalcaemia. For example, in chronic renal failure, secondary hyperparathyroidism can lead to hypercalcaemia and metastatic calcification; in the eye, such deposition of calcium can occur in the conjunctiva or cornea as band keratopathy. By contrast, dystrophic calcification occurs in normocalcaemia, typically in necrotic or hyalinised tissue. An example of this is a phthisical eye.

    Calcium is usually deposited in the form of hydroxyapatite crystals.

    Band keratopathy is non-specific and involves calcification of the subepithelium, Bowman's layer and the superficial stroma in the interpalpebral cornea. It can occur in otherwise healthy eyes as a senile degenerative phenomenon, or secondary to hypercalcaemia, or due to ocular causes such as chronic anterior segment inflammation (e.g. chronic uveitis).

93. **D Neutrophil activation**

    Amyloid deposition is associated with some chronic inflammatory disorders, such as rheumatoid arthritis.

    Giant cells are transformed fused macrophages and occur in chronic inflammatory disorders such as chalazion, giant cell arteritis and granulomatous conditions such as sarcoid and tuberculosis.

    Necrosis is a feature of tuberculosis, actinomycosis and syphilis.

    Neutrophil activation and the subsequent respiratory burst are typical features of acute inflammation, whereas the cellular infiltrate in chronic inflammation tends to be predominantly macrophages and lymphocytes.

94. C Förster–Fuchs' spot

Bergmeister's papilla is a cone-like fibrous structure that is sometimes observed at the optic nerve head as a remnant of the hyaloid artery. The central retinal artery is formed from the proximal segment of the hyaloid artery. Mittendorf's dot is a small opacity that is sometimes observed on the posterior lens capsule at the point of anterior attachment of the hyaloid artery. Both Bergmeister's papilla and Mittendorf's dot are benign variants, as opposed to pathological persistent foetal vasculature. Förster–Fuchs' spot is a pigmented macular scar associated with pathological myopia.

95. B Betaxolol

Betaxolol is an adrenoceptor antagonist selective for the β_1 receptor. It lowers intraocular pressure by reducing aqueous production by the ciliary body and has no effect on outflow. It has a lower rate of bronchospasm as this side effect is β_2-mediated.

Timolol (the most commonly-used topical anti-glaucoma agent globally) and levobunolol are both non-selective β antagonists. Apraclonidine is an α_2 agonist.

96. D Metabolic acidosis

Carbonic anhydrase catalyses the production of carbonic acid from water and carbon dioxide, which then dissociates into hydrogen ions and bicarbonate, as follows:

$$H_2O + CO_2 \leftrightarrow H_2CO_3 \leftrightarrow H^+ + HCO_3^-$$

Carbonic anhydrase inhibition, e.g. by an oral agent such as acetazolamide, slows this reaction and can result in a metabolic acidosis by increasing renal excretion of bicarbonate. A side effect of acetazolamide is potassium depletion with the risk of hypokalaemia.

The effect of carbonic anhydrase inhibition on the eye is to lower intraocular pressure, by causing reduced aqueous secretion from the non-pigmented ciliary epithelium.

97. D Pilocarpine 0.1%

The likely diagnosis is Adie's pupil, which most commonly affects young women. This affects the parasympathetic supply to the iris via the ciliary ganglion. Loss of postganglionic nerve fibres results in denervation hypersensitivity, such that the iris sphincter becomes supersensitive to dilute pilocarpine (e.g. 0.1%). Pilocarpine is a muscarinic agonist that, in normal eyes, requires concentrations of approximately 1% or greater to cause miosis.

98. B They affect gene transcription

Corticosteroids bind to specific intracellular receptors in the cytoplasm, which then translocate to the nucleus and affect gene transcription (thyroid hormones also act in a similar manner). As the main anti-inflammatory actions of corticosteroids are brought about by changes in gene transcription, they can take hours or days to develop. An important component of this is reducing the transcription of the gene for cyclooxygenase-2, which results in decreased prostanoid production. Steroids also exert non-genomic effects, which have a more rapid onset and are the subject of ongoing research.

99. B Inhalational anaesthetic agents are associated with a rise in intraocular pressure

Inhalational anaesthetic agents tend to reduce intraocular pressure (IOP), as do all intravenous induction agents except ketamine. Intravenous induction agents include propofol, thiopentone and etomidate.

Both atropine and, more commonly, glycopyrrolate (the active moiety of glycopyrronium bromide) are anticholinergics used to blunt the oculocardiac reflex during eye surgery. Commonly triggered during squint surgery, the oculocardiac reflex results in vagally-mediated bradycardia which may progress to asystole.

Suxamethonium produces depolarising neuromuscular blockade and is used to paralyse skeletal muscle during general anaesthesia. Suxamethonium causes a rise in IOP, possibly mediated by a combination of extraocular muscle fasciculation and choroidal vasodilatation.

100. B Liver

By far the most common site of metastasis from choroidal melanoma is the liver (approximately 90%), followed by lung, bone and skin. Patients with choroidal melanoma should be monitored with regular liver imaging. In the UK and Europe, this typically involves an ultrasound of the liver every 6 months for 10 years, followed up with CT or MRI if a suspicious lesion is detected.

Systemic metastases generally spread via the blood, as the uvea does not have lymphatics. Only 2–4% of patients have metastastic disease at diagnosis.

101. B Heparin may cause paradoxical thrombosis, due to thrombocytosis

Unfractionated heparin (UFH) is the term given to the originally discovered substance, but shorter heparin fragments, known as low-molecular weight heparin (LMWH), have several advantages as anticoagulants.

UFH potentiates the action of antithrombin, which inactivates several clotting factors but principally thrombin and factor Xa. It also inhibits platelet aggregation by fibrin. LMWH preferentially affects factor Xa, with much less effect on thrombin.

Side effects of heparin include: bleeding; thrombocytopenia (which may paradoxically cause thrombosis); osteoporosis with prolonged use; and hypoaldosteronism, with consequent hyperkalaemia.

Heparins are strongly acidic. Protamine is a strongly basic protein which reverses the effects of UFH, and can partially reverse some LMWHs.

102. A Atropine 1%

Atropine 1% induces mydriasis lasting up to 7 days (and sometimes longer), and reaches its maximum mydriatic effect after 30–40 minutes. Cyclopentolate 1% induces mydriasis lasting up to 24 hours and reaches its maximum mydriatic effect after 20–60 minutes. Homatropine 2% induces mydriasis lasting 6 hours to 4 days and reaches its maximum mydriatic effect after 10–30 minutes. Tropicamide 1% induces mydriasis lasting 4–6 hours, and reaches its maximum mydriatic effect after 15–30 minutes.

Darker irides generally take longer to attain the maximum mydriatic effect than lighter irides. Selection of an appropriate mydriatic should take into account the duration of action required (note that the duration of cycloplegia is not equal to the duration of mydriasis).

103. A Chloramphenicol

Chloramphenicol has the rare but serious haematological side effects of bone marrow suppression and aplastic anaemia. The risk of these is negligible with topical chloramphenicol, but more significant when given systemically. Due to these safety concerns, systemic chloramphenicol is very rarely used in the developed world.

104. D It requires phosphorylation to become active

Aciclovir is a guanosine derivative that requires phosphorylation by thymidine kinase as the first step in its activation. The viral form of thymidine kinase is far more effective at performing this than the human (host cell) form, meaning that the drug is principally activated in infected cells. It is then further phosphorylated to its active form, aciclovir triphosphate, by host cell kinases.

Aciclovir inhibits viral DNA polymerase and hence viral replication. The monophosphate form is also incorporated into viral DNA, leading to chain termination. Its effects are highly specific to herpes simplex and herpes zoster (varicella zoster) viruses, with herpes simplex being the more susceptible of the two. It is frequently used in ophthalmology to treat keratitis and uveitis caused by these viruses. Aciclovir also has some (lesser) activity against Epstein–Barr and cytomegalovirus.

105. D Tay–Sachs disease

Tay–Sachs disease is an autosomal recessive condition characterised by progressive neurodegeneration caused by accumulation of GM2 ganglioside molecules. It results from mutations of the *HEXA* gene on chromosome 15 which encodes a component of a lysosomal enzyme. These mutations typically involve insertions, deletions and point mutations.

By contrast, the other three disorders (as well as fragile X syndrome and Friedreich's ataxia) are caused by triplet repeat expansions. These are abnormal expansions of a trinucleotide sequence leading to mis-function or non-function of the resulting proteins, and/or aggregation of abnormal protein leading to disease. Diseases caused by triplet repeat expansions are generally autosomal dominant and have an earlier onset and increased severity with increased size of the triplet repeat expansion. With each generation the repeat sequence typically expands, leading to the phenomenon of genetic anticipation.

106. B Full-field electroretinogram

A full-field (Ganzfeld) electroretinogram (ERG) measures the electrical response of the retina as a whole when stimulated by a bright flash of light. By contrast, the multifocal ERG is a newer technique that allows more localised testing of the retina, by stimulating multiple retinal areas independently and simultaneously.

The electrooculogram (EOG) measures the standing potential between the front and back of the eye. Visual-evoked potentials are a measure of the electrical response of the visual cortex to a changing visual stimulus (e.g. change in pattern, luminance or contrast).

107. C Aortic stenosis results in reduced stroke volume

Regarding cardiac output:

- Cardiac output = stroke volume × heart rate
- Stroke volume = end-diastolic volume − end systolic volume

Stroke volume is affected by preload, afterload and myocardial contractility. Starling's law describes an important cardiac homeostatic mechanism, where the force of contraction of the myocardium is proportional to the initial muscle fibre length. Within limits, this means that an increase in preload increases stroke volume, whereas an increase in afterload (which results in increased end systolic volume) decreases stroke volume.

Aortic stenosis decreases stroke volume by increasing afterload, whilst amyloid infiltration of the myocardium can reduce ventricular compliance and impair ventricular filling.

108. D The oxygen binding affinity of haemoglobin is reduced by acidity

Haemoglobin is composed of:

- Haem, a derivative of porphyrin containing ferrous (Fe^{2+}) iron (oxidation to ferric or Fe^{3+} iron occurs in methaemoglobinaemia)
- Globin, which consists of four polypeptide chains (each with a haem moeity)

In adult haemoglobin, HbA, there are two α polypeptide chains and two β chains, whereas foetal HbF contains two α chains and two γ chains. Foetal haemoglobin has a higher affinity for oxygen.

The oxygen–haemoglobin dissociation curve is shifted to the right (i.e. reduced oxygen binding affinity) by increasing acidity and pCO_2 (the Bohr effect), temperature and 2,3-DPG.

Thalassaemia results in reduced synthesis of normal globin chains, whereas sickle cell anaemia is characterised by abnormal β chain production.

109. C Melanin granules and phagosomes are abundant in the cytoplasm

Melanin pigment granules and phagosomes are abundant in the cytoplasm of retinal pigment epithelium (RPE) cells. Melanin has a role in protection from light scatter, light damage and oxidative stress. It is the principal absorber of laser light during panretinal photocoagulation.

Tight junctions (zonulae occludentes) between RPE cells are responsible for maintaining the blood–retinal barrier, not Bruch's membrane.

Each RPE cell interdigitates with many photoreceptors; the ratio of photoreceptors to RPE cells varies across the retina but is approximately 45:1 at the posterior pole.

Opsins are synthesised by photoreceptors, not the RPE. The RPE is responsible for the regeneration of 11-*cis*-retinal.

110. A 2.5 µL/min

Aqueous humour is produced at an average rate of approximately 2.5 µL/min. Production is usually slightly higher in the morning (around 3 µL/min) and slightly lower overnight (around 1.5 µL/min), and approximately 2.5 µL/min throughout the rest of the day. There is a slow decline in the rate of production with age.

111. A Erect, virtual, displaced towards the apex

Triangular prisms form an image that is erect, virtual and displaced towards the apex of the prism. This is best seen in **Figure 3.4** below.

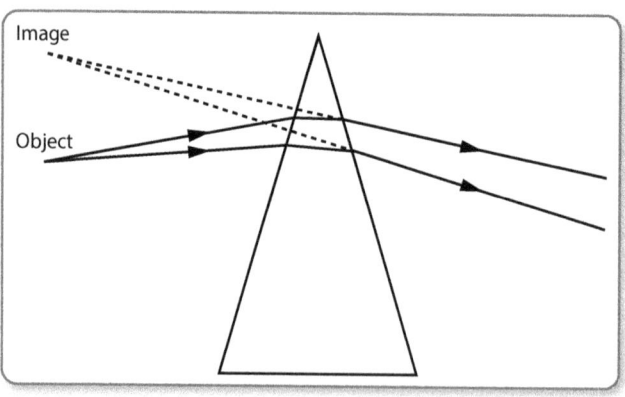

Figure 3.4 Image formation by a triangular prism.

Answers: SBAs

112. C 2, 3 and 5

The layered inputs to the lateral geniculate nucleus are arranged so that ipsilateral fibres arrive in layers 2, 3 and 5 while contralateral fibres arrive in layers 1, 4 and 6. The reason for this division is not entirely clear. The fibres are arranged in a topographic pattern that is consistent between layers. It is interesting to note that although both the retina and the lateral geniculate nucleus have a topographic organisation, the optic nerve itself does not.

113. D Vagus nerve

The innervation of the pharyngeal arches is shown in **Table 3.10**.

Note that the pharyngeal arches are numbered according to their evolutionary precursors in fish, hence the absence of a 5th pharyngeal arch.

Table 3.10 Innervation of pharyngeal arches	
Pharyngeal arch	Cranial nerve
1	Trigeminal (V) – maxillary and mandibular branches
2	Facial (VII)
3	Glossopharyngeal (IX)
4	Vagus (X) – superior laryngeal branch
6	Vagus (X) – recurrent laryngeal branch

114. B Both focal lines are in front of the retina

In compound astigmatism, both focal lines are either in front of (myopic) or behind (hypermetropic) the retina. This is in contrast to 'simple' astigmatism, in which one of the focal lines lies on the retina. In mixed astigmatism, the focal lines straddle the retina.

Note that this description of astigmatism is based on the focal lines of the principal meridians in relation to the retina. Astigmatism can also be described in terms of the axis of the principal meridians of the eye, e.g. regular versus irregular, 'with' versus 'against' the rule.

115. D 98%

The uveal tract has an extremely high rate of blood flow, which is greater per unit volume than most other tissues in the body, including the kidney. As such some 98% of the ocular circulation passes through the uveal tract.

116. B Pretectal nucleus

Some 90% of optic nerve fibres travel to the lateral geniculate nucleus, with the remaining 10% travelling along the medial root of the optic tract to subcortical targets. **Table 3.11** provides a summary of key subcortical targets and their principal functions.

Table 3.11 Subcortical targets of optic nerve fibres	
Subcortical target	Principal functions
Superior colliculus	Directing visual attention; auditory/visual integration; grasp reflex; coordination of head and eye movements
Suprachiasmatic nucleus	Circadian rhythm
Pretectal nuclei	Pupillary light reflex
Pulvinar nucleus	Visual attention and integration of visual input with motor responses
Parvocellular reticular formation	Arousal function

117. A Auditory/visual integration

Intrinsically photosensitive retinal ganglion cells (ipRGCs) contain the photopigment melanopsin, which has a peak spectral sensitivity in the blue–violet range. 5 subtypes of ipRGCs have been identified at present, along with a growing range of recognised functions. Studies on patients without rod or cone function have demonstrated roles for ipRGCs in modulating circadian rhythm, sleep cycle regulation and the pupillary light reflex, and possibly a role in conscious vision as a detector of mean brightness. The receptive fields of ipRGCs are too diffuse to imply a role in auditory/visual integration.

118. C They can only carry a limited amount of genetic material

Viral vectors are highly efficient at transduction, and can be modified to prevent them replicating and causing disease. Even after such engineering they retain the ability to target and enter cells.

The two principal disadvantages are as follows:

- They can only carry a limited amount of genetic material, so some genes are too large
- They are immunogenic

119. D 2.5 µm

The standard error of the mean (SEM) is a measure of how good an estimate the mean of a sample from a population is of the true mean of that population. It is calculated using the following formula:

$$SEM = \frac{S}{\sqrt{n}}$$

where S is the standard deviation of the sample (in this case 25 µm); and n is the sample size (in this case 100).

Therefore:

$$SEM = \frac{25 \text{ µm}}{\sqrt{100}} = \frac{25 \text{ µm}}{10} = 2.5 \text{ µm}$$

It is worth noting that since n will always be >1, the standard error of the mean will always be smaller than the standard deviation.

120. C Greater petrosal nerve

While the foramen ovale sometimes transmits the lesser petrosal nerve from the middle cranial fossa, it does not transmit the greater petrosal nerve. A good mnemonic for structures which can pass through the foramen ovale is:

O – Otic ganglion (typically lies just inferior to the foramen ovale)

V – V3 (mandibular branch of the trigeminal nerve)

A – Accessory meningeal artery

L – Lesser petrosal nerve (this may also pass via other small foraminae between the foramen ovale and foramen spinosum)

E – Emissary veins

Answers: CRQs

1. **Answer**

   (a) The epidermis

   Feedback
   The cutis is the anatomical term for the outer layers of the skin, and is composed of the superficial epidermis and the deeper dermis. The basal cells are proliferating keratinocytes immediately superficial to the basement membrane of the epidermis.

   (b) Slide B shows a micronodular basal cell carcinoma (BCC) and is more concerning than slide A, which shows a nodular or solid BCC. Micronodular BCCs are more aggressive, and often have subclinical spread beyond their macroscopic boundaries, making it harder to determine clear margins during excision.

   (1 mark for identifying slide B as the more concerning; 1 mark for justifying with increased risk of subclinical spread)

   Feedback
   There are a number of histological subtypes of BCC. The four that are most important to be able to recognise as an ophthalmologist are: nodular (or solid) BCCs, like in slide A, which are well circumscribed with clear peripheral palisading and are easily excised; superficial BCCs, which appear histologically as lobules localised to the dermal–epidermal junction; infiltrative (or morphoeic) BCCs, which grow aggressively in strands with reduced peripheral palisading and an indistinct border; and micronodular BCCs, like in slide B, where there are multiple small nodular aggregates of tumour.

   Both infiltrative BCCs and micronodular BCCs have an increased tendency for subclinical spread, and caution should be taken to ensure clear margins.

   (c) Local invasion

   Feedback
   Basal cell carcinomas (BCCs) almost never metastasise (reported incidence of less than 0.1%), but they can invade local tissues aggressively. Perivascular and perineural invasion have been reported with the most aggressive BCCs.

   (d) Whether all margins are clear and the tumours are completely excised

   Feedback
   It is very important to confirm that the lesions are histologically completely excised, particularly in the case of the micronodular BCC in slide B. Recurrence in the periocular area carries the risk of orbital invasion, which may require exenteration.

(e) Any two of:
- Fair skin/Caucasian
- Accumulated sun exposure (therefore age indirectly)
- Immunosuppression
- Male gender
- Previous history of skin cancer
- Chronic skin infection/inflammation
- Radiation exposure
- Arsenic exposure

(*1 mark for each up to 2 marks*)

Feedback
The two principal risk factors for basal cell carcinomas (BCCs) are fair skin and accumulated sun exposure. For this reason they predominantly occur in older Caucasian individuals and on sun-exposed surfaces. An increasing number of younger individuals are developing BCCs, most probably due to increased sun exposure and the use of sunbeds.

(f) Superficial basal cell carcinoma (BCC)

Feedback
Imiquimod is an immune response modulator and has been shown to stimulate apoptosis in BCC cells. It has been demonstrated to be an effective topical treatment for superficial BCCs with histological clearance rates of 82–90%. Some studies have also reported the use of imiquimod on nodular BCCs, and it has been demonstrated as a relatively effective treatment in circumstances where surgery may not be appropriate. However, surgery remains the mainstay of treatment for nodular BCCs, especially in the periocular region. Inoperable tumours with significant morbidity may be treated with systemic Hedgehog pathway inhibitors such as Vismodegib, although this is not currently recommended by NICE, partially on grounds of cost-effectiveness.

(g) Any two of:
- Gorlin–Goltz syndrome (or basal cell naevus syndrome; nevoid basal cell carcinoma syndrome; Gorlin syndrome)
- Xeroderma pigmentosum
- Albinism
- Bazex syndrome (Bazex–Dupré–Christol syndrome)

(*1 mark for each entity up to 2 marks: any of the above terminologies may be used*)

Feedback
Gorlin–Goltz syndrome is an autosomal dominant condition characterised by multiple basal cell carcinomas (BCCs) at an early age. It is also associated with a number of craniofacial and musculoskeletal abnormalities, and certain other neoplasms and hamartomas.

Xeroderma pigmentosum is an autosomal recessive disorder characterised by extreme sensitivity to UV light. Affected individuals are susceptible to developing all skin cancers and frequently develop multiple BCCs at an early age.

Albinism is also usually autosomal recessive, and affected individuals are at an increased risk of all skin cancers due to their lack of melanin.

Bazex–Dupré–Christol syndrome is a rare X-linked dominant disorder of hair follicles which is associated with early onset of multiple facial BCCs (not to be confused with acrokeratosis neoplastica, also sometimes called Bazex syndrome, which is an unrelated rare psoriasiform dermatosis associated with squamous cell carcinoma of the upper respiratory and gastrointestinal tract).

2. **Answer**

(a) $F_2 = \dfrac{F_1}{1 - dF_1}$

Where F_2 is the power of the new lens required at 7 mm; F_1 is the power of the original lens (10 dioptres); d is the distance the lens is moved towards the eye in metres (0.005 metres)

$$F_2 = \dfrac{10}{1 - 0.05}$$

$$= \dfrac{10}{0.95}$$

$$= 10.526$$

Therefore, a 10.5 dioptre lens would be appropriate *(1 mark for correct formula, 1 mark for correct calculation)*

Feedback
With this type of calculation remember that the units of distance are metres, although the back vertex distance is generally expressed in millimetres. It is also vital to get the sign of d correct: it is positive if the lens is moved towards the eye and negative if the lens is moved away from the eye. Remember that calculators are not usually allowed in the examination and you must be prepared to do long division on paper at least to this level of complexity.

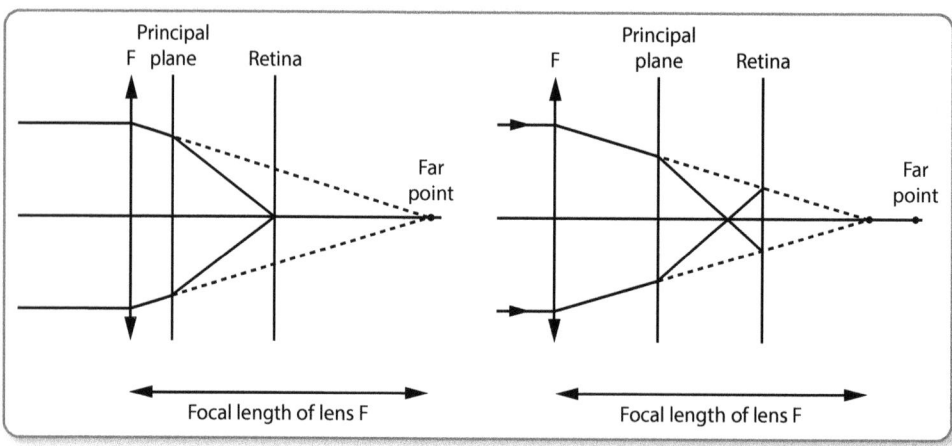

(b) Diagram of convex lens moving away from the eye

(*2 marks per ray diagram: must show lens, principal plane and retina; second diagram must show crossing of rays or a focal point in front of the retina*)

(c) Pin-cushion distortion

Feedback
High powered convex lenses produce pin-cushion distortion, whereas high powered concave lenses cause barrel distortion.

(d) 2 dioptres base out

Feedback

$$P = F \times D$$

Where P is the induced prismatic power in prism dioptres; F is the power of the decentred lens in dioptres; and D is the decentration in centimetres.

The easiest way to determine the direction of prism power is to imagine convex lenses as two prisms attached base to base and concave lenses as two prisms attached apex to apex. Thus, when a convex lens is decentred the base of the lens is always towards the optical centre, i.e. in the same direction as the lens is moved, whereas the opposite is true for concave lenses.

(e)
- Ring scotoma
- 'Jack-in-the-box' phenomenon

(*1 mark each*)

Feedback
The prismatic effect of strong convex lenses such as those prescribed for aphakia cause a ring scotoma around the edge of the spectacle lens. Objects can appear or disappear as the patient moves their eyes or head (and therefore their ring scotoma). This is known as the 'jack-in-the-box' phenomenon.

3. **Answer**

(a) Thyroid stimulating hormone (TSH) receptor antibodies (TRAb)

Feedback
The condition most commonly associated with thyroid eye disease is Graves' disease, in which stimulatory TSH receptor antibodies cause hyperthyroidism. The antibodies are thought to cross-react with orbital fibroblast antigens, resulting in the activation of inflammatory cascades and development of orbitopathy.

TSH receptor antibodies are the most likely antibody to be positive in thyroid eye disease, but anti-thyroid peroxidase (anti-TPO) and anti-thyroglobulin antibodies may also be detected.

Hashimoto's thyroiditis is also associated with thyroid eye disease, but the association is far weaker than with Graves' disease.

In the scenario presented, the ophthalmic diagnosis is clear from the clinical presentation and thyroid function. However, thyroid and ocular manifestations of thyroid eye disease do not always occur simultaneously, and in cases where the thyroid function is normal, positive thyroid autoantibodies can support the diagnosis.

(b) Any four of the following:

- Sinus tachycardia
- Atrial fibrillation
- Tremor
- Warm, moist peripheries
- Palmar erythema
- Hair loss
- Muscle weakness
- Pretibial myxoedema
- Thyroid acropachy (digital clubbing also accepted)

Feedback

Systemic clinical features of hyperthyroidism are listed in **Table 3.12** below.

Table 3.12 Systemic clinical features of hyperthyroidism	
Symptoms of hyperthyroidism	**Signs of hyperthyroidism**

• Palpitations
• Anxiety, altered mood, insomnia
• Sweating, heat intolerance
• Dyspnoea
• Weight loss +/− increased appetite
• Diarrhoea
• Amenorrhoea
• Loss of libido
	• Sinus tachycardia
	• Atrial fibrillation
	• Tremor
	• Warm, moist peripheries
	• Palmar erythema
	• Hair loss
	• Muscle weakness
	• Specific to Graves:
	  – Pretibial myxoedema
	  – Thyroid acropachy

(c) A pregnancy test should be performed. The two most likely explanations for the amenorrhoea are pregnancy or hyperthyroidism. If this patient is pregnant, this is likely to influence the treatment options for both her hyperthyroidism and her thyroid eye disease.

Feedback

Amenorrhoea, or more commonly oligomenorrhoea, occurs in hyperthyroidism. This is related to more widespread endocrine disturbance including changes in sex-hormone-binding globulin. Equally, this patient may be pregnant, and autoimmune thyroid disease is more common in pregnancy.

The mainstay of medical treatment for hyperthyroidism is systemic anti-thyroid medication. The choice of drug may be altered if the patient is pregnant, and radioiodine is contraindicated in pregnancy.

Lastly, this patient is a smoker, and smoking cessation is particularly important both in pregnancy and in patients with thyroid eye disease, in whom it worsens the severity and outcome of the disease.

(d)

- Orthoptist
- Endocrinologist

Feedback
This patient is hyperthyroid and has diplopia, and so multidisciplinary input from endocrinology and orthoptics is vital in her care. The severity of thyroid eye disease is reduced by scrupulous control of thyroid function, in addition to the implications for her systemic health. Progressive restriction of eye movements can reflect increased disease activity, and when the disease is 'burnt out', squint surgery may be of benefit. Orthoptic monitoring may include ancillary testing such as a uniocular field of fixation, field of binocular single vision and Hess chart.

(e)

- Optic neuropathy
- Exposure keratopathy

Feedback
The two principal sight-threatening complications in thyroid eye disease (TED) are optic neuropathy and exposure keratopathy. Monitoring of TED includes careful assessment of optic nerve function, lid closure and corneal integrity so that these can be detected promptly to prevent or minimise visual loss.

Acute optic neuropathy is managed with high-dose systemic corticosteroids, sometimes with the addition of other immunosuppressants or radiotherapy, and in cases unresponsive to steroids, with emergency orbital decompression.

The management of exposure keratopathy depends on the severity, and may include lubricants, lid taping, tarsorrhaphy, systemic steroids/immuno-suppression, and rarely emergency orbital decompression.

4. Answer

(a) The structures labelled A and B are:

A: Superior orbital fissure

B: (Lesser wing of the) sphenoid

(½ mark each)

(b)

The nerves labelled C, which pass outside the common tendinous ring, are the lacrimal nerve (V1), frontal nerve (V1) and trochlear nerve (IV). The nerve labelled D is the optic nerve *(½ mark each)*

(c)

The nerves labelled E, which pass within the common tendinous ring, are the superior division of III, the nasociliary nerve (V1), the inferior division of III, and the abducens nerve (VI) *(½ mark each)*

(d) The structures labelled F and G are the superior and inferior ophthalmic veins, respectively *(½ mark each)*

(e) The muscles labelled H to M and their motor nerve supply are:

H – Lateral rectus: Abducens nerve (VI)

I – Superior rectus: Oculomotor nerve (III)

J – Levator palpebrae superioris: Oculomotor nerve (III)

K – Superior oblique: Trochlear nerve (IV)

L – Medial rectus: Oculomotor nerve (III)

M – Inferior rectus: Oculomotor nerve (III)

(½ mark each)

(f) Sudden visual loss in the ipsilateral eye with ocular ischaemia

Feedback
The vessel labelled N is the ophthalmic artery. TIAs commonly affect the internal carotid artery territory, including the ophthalmic artery (causing amaurosis fugax). They are typically embolic, with atherosclerosis of the ipsilateral carotid artery. Chronic hypoperfusion of the eye may also result from carotid atherosclerosis and cause ocular ischaemic syndrome.

Ophthalmic artery occlusion results in occlusion of both the retinal and choroidal circulations. This is distinct from a central retinal artery occlusion (CRAO), where only the inner retina becomes ischaemic, but the two conditions present in a similar manner with acute visual loss. In ophthalmic artery occlusion, the visual loss tends to be even more severe with little or no light perception. Furthermore, as the choroidal circulation is also affected, the cherry red spot seen in CRAO is not visible.

5. Answer

(a) Any two of:

- Hard exudates (circinate exudates also correct)
- Microaneurysms (or dot haemorrhages)
- Blot haemorrhages
- Cotton wool spot

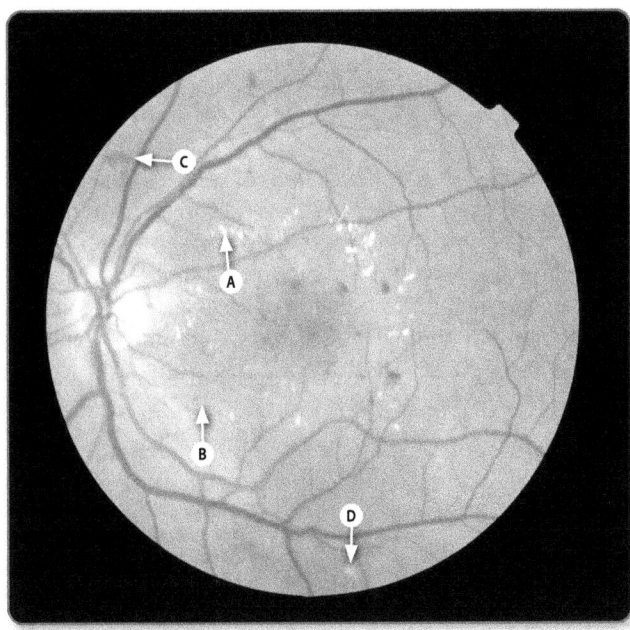

A – Hard exudates. When these are found in a circular distribution around an area of haemorrhage, these may be referred to circinate exudates
B – Microaneurysms or dot haemorrhages
C – Blot haemorrhages
D – Cotton wool spot

Feedback
An example of each of the fundal signs is indicated in the figure above.

(b) Optical coherence tomography (OCT) scan of the macula

(c) Diabetic macular oedema *(centre-involving macular oedema, or clinically-significant macular oedema, are both also valid. Only ½ mark if diabetes not specifically mentioned)*

Feedback
The presence of macular oedema, together with the fundus findings of retinal haemorrhage, hard exudates and cotton wool spots, are very suggestive of diabetic macular oedema. This is caused by breakdown of the inner blood–retinal barrier with extensive leakage from capillaries and microaneurysms. Initially, the oedema occurs between the inner nuclear and outer plexiform layers, but with increasing fluid accumulation the other retinal layers become involved, which, at the fovea, gives a characteristic cystoid appearance.

(d) Intravitreal injection of anti-VEGF (anti-vascular endothelial growth factor):

Upregulation of vascular endothelial growth factor (VEGF) is implicated in the breakdown of the blood–retinal barrier and increased capillary permeability, which lead to macular oedema. In the eye, the principal subtype is VEGF-A which acts on tyrosine kinase-linked receptors (e.g. VEGFR-2). Other growth factors have been implicated in diabetic retinopathy, such as angiopoietin 2 (ANG-2), with associated vascular endothelial disruption and development of macular oedema. Intravitreal injections of monoclonal antibodies against VEGF (e.g. ranibizumab, bevacizumab), VEGF inhibitors (e.g. aflibercept, a recombinant fusion protein which binds VEGF), or monoclonal antibodies which target both VEGF and ANG-2 (e.g. faricimab) block these actions, and can stabilise or improve vision by reducing macular oedema.

Macular laser (grid or focal):

Laser to areas of macular oedema, either to focal areas of leakage (focal laser) or diffusely (grid laser) has been used for decades to reduce macular oedema. Although the primary effect of laser in this context is a thermal burn to the retinal pigment epithelium (RPE), the exact mechanism by which it reduces oedema is debated. Proposed mechanisms include stimulation of vascular endothelial cells and proliferation of retinal pigment epithelial cells, improving both the inner and outer blood-retinal barriers, respectively. The area within 500 μm of the fovea is avoided as this is likely to cause visual loss.

(1 mark for each correct treatment option, with 1 mark for a sensible mode of action containing elements of the above. ½ mark only for: conservative measures of improving glycaemic and hypertensive control; intravitreal steroid; vitrectomy. No marks for panretinal photocoagulation)

Feedback
Whilst macular laser is still used to treat macular oedema in diabetes, intravitreal anti-VEGF injections have been shown to be superior to laser alone for centre-involving oedema and form the mainstay of treatment.

Tightening of glycaemic and hypertensive control is an important measure in reducing the development of sight-threatening disease, but once symptomatic centre-involving macular oedema (involving the fovea) has developed, such as in this case, intervention in the form of anti-VEGF injections or laser is required.

Other treatments such as intravitreal steroid and vitrectomy are sometimes used in the treatment of macular oedema, but are not typically first-line treatments.

(e) Any two of:

- Wet age-related macular degeneration (AMD)
- Cystoid macular oedema (a recognised cause of CMO is also acceptable, e.g. post-operative inflammation following intraocular surgery, uveitis, retinal vein occlusion)
- Hypertensive retinopathy
 (1 mark each)

6. Answer

(a) Left sixth cranial nerve *(1 mark for correct nerve, 1 mark for laterality)*

Feedback
The Hess chart shows left lateral rectus underaction, with corresponding right medial rectus overaction. The nerve supply to the lateral rectus is from the ipsilateral sixth cranial nerve (cf. fourth cranial nerve, whose nucleus supplies the contralateral superior oblique).

(b) Possible aetiologies for sixth cranial nerve palsies include:
- Microvascular ischaemia
- Tumours (e.g. skull base meningioma)
- Trauma
- Stroke
- Vasculitis (e.g. GCA)
- Demyelination
- Raised intracranial pressure (commonly bilateral)
- Gradenigo syndrome (rare in the era of modern antibiotics)

(1 mark each, up to 3 marks)

Feedback

The most common cause of unilateral sixth cranial nerve palsy is microvascular ischaemia, for which diabetes and hypertension are important risk factors. There is a high chance of full recovery within weeks to months.

(c) The pons

(d) A 30 prism dioptre base out Fresnel prism (to right or left lens of glasses). Alternatively this can be split, e.g. into 15 prism dioptres base out to each eye.

(1 mark for single base out prism, 1 mark for split prisms)

(e)

Fresnel prism diagram

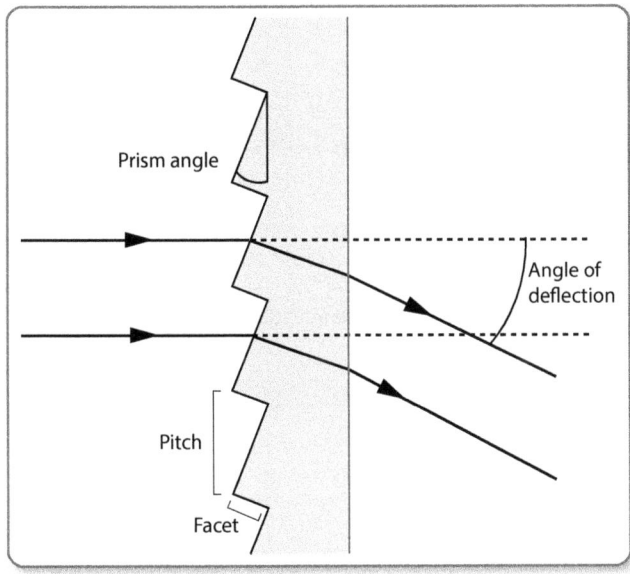

(1 mark for correct illustration of multiple prisms, 1 mark for deflection of parallel light rays)

7. Answer

(a)
- A: Optic vesicle
- B: Otic placode
- C: Pharyngeal arches
- D: Heart bulge

(1 mark for each correctly labelled structure)

Feedback
This is a diagram of the developing embryo at 27 days. The optic vesicle (A) can be observed with the otic placode (B) lying caudal to it. The pharyngeal arches (C), with the pharyngeal clefts between, emerge rostral to the larger heart bulge (D).

(b)
- A: Optic stalk
- B: Optic vesicle
- C: Retinal disk
- D: Lens placode

(1 mark for each correctly labelled structure)

Feedback
This is a diagram of the developing eye at 27 days. The optic stalk (A) connects the optic vesicle (B) to the neural ectoderm of the prosencephalon. The retinal disk (C) is formed as a circular thickening of the neural ectoderm, and will later form the neural retina. The lens placode (D) is formed as a thickening of the surface ectoderm.

(c) The subretinal space *(1 mark)*

Feedback
The space indicated is the cavity of the optic vesicle, also known as the optic ventricle. As the eye develops, this will become the subretinal space.

(d) 5 weeks *(1 mark)*

Feedback
The lens vesicle typically separates from the surface ectoderm by the start of day 36, i.e. after 5 weeks.

8. Answer

(a) Coma aberration

Feedback
Coma aberration is a variant of spherical aberration which occurs with light originating from points away from the principal axis. Light rays passing through the lens periphery are deviated more than those passing through the central portion of the lens. This consequently leads to a composite image that is elongated like the tail of a comet.

(b) Keratoconus

Feedback
Patients with keratoconus experience a number of simple and higher order optical aberrations, and in particular, they are susceptible to coma and coma-like aberrations.

(c) Chromatic aberration

(d)

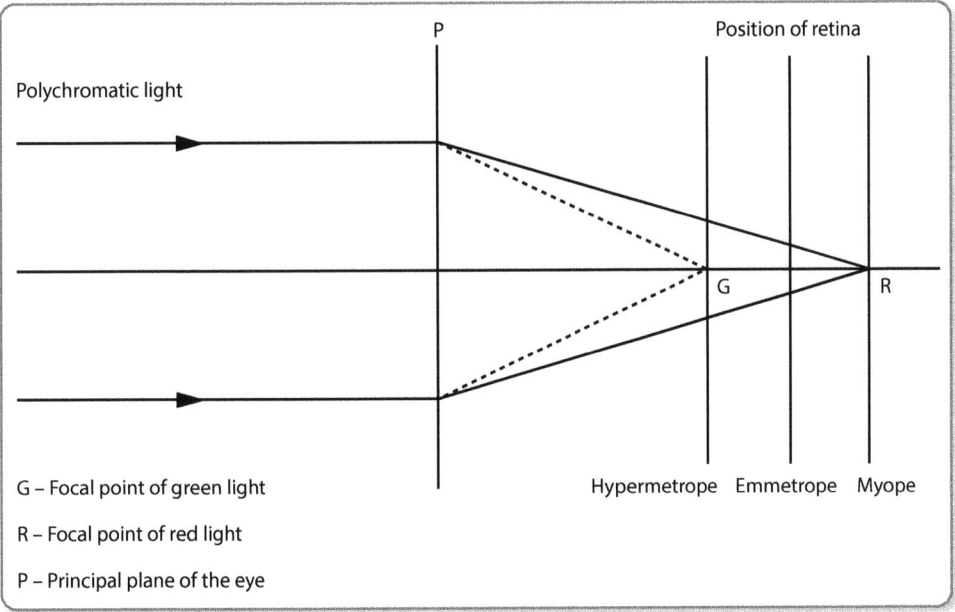

(1 mark for each correctly labelled point – the retinal positions do not have to be exactly at the focal points of red and green light, but should be close, as the duochrome test is utilised for small refinements in prescription)

(e) A colour blind patient should be asked whether the letters are clearer on the upper or lower row.

Feedback
The optics remain the same regardless of whether the patient can tell which colour is red and which is green.

(f) Spherical aberration

Feedback
Under normal circumstances the iris acts as a 'stop' to occlude the passage of light through the periphery of the lens, thus reducing spherical aberration. When the pupil is dilated there is a dramatic increase in spherical aberration and a consequent decrease in visual acuity.

9. Answer

(a) In the inferotemporal retinal vasculature there are focal areas of bunching and dilatation of the capillaries. Also, there are ghost vessels in the inferotemporal venous system.

(1 mark for each abnormality)

Feedback
A red-free fundus image is taken prior to the injection of fluorescein dye.

The appearance is suspicious of new retinal vessels inferotemporally, but the fundus fluorescein angiogram (FFA) findings will help to confirm this. The venous ghost vessels are suggestive of previous vein occlusion. The small focal areas of lighter pigmentation in the surrounding retina, which are particularly visible in the inferotemporal macula, are laser scars.

(b)

1. Abnormal new vessels (neovascularisation).
2. Laser scars.

(1 mark for each cause)

Feedback
There is diffuse hyperfluorescence around the capillaries of the inferotemporal retina, which in the peripheral retina increases dramatically in size and intensity over time in a pattern consistent with leakage of dye due to retinal neovascularisation.

The key features of leakage are an increase in the size and intensity of the hyperfluorescence over time. The appearance of the vessels in the inferotemporal area on the red-free image was suspicious of new vessels, and the pattern of dye leakage confirms this.

Leakage can be due to incompetence of one of the two blood–retinal barriers (inner/outer), and may come from the retinal circulation, such as in neovascularisation or cystoid macular oedema, or the choroidal circulation (e.g. wet AMD).

There are multiple small areas of focal hyperfluorescence, which appear early and increase slightly in intensity but not in size. This is consistent with transmitted choroidal fluorescence due to a retinal pigment epithelium (RPE) window defect caused by laser scars.

Hyperfluorescence due to a window defect is typically caused by RPE atrophy, which unmasks the normal choroidal fluorescence. A key differentiating feature is that it appears very early, whereas hyperfluorescence due to staining with dye (e.g. drusen, disciform scars) appears late.

(c) Right inferotemporal branch retinal vein occlusion

Feedback
The findings of new vessels (neovascularisation) and capillary dropout indicate ischaemia. Whilst diabetic retinopathy is a common cause of new vessels, the

segmental distribution in this case combined with the venous ghost vessels make the most likely aetiology a branch retinal vein occlusion. The distribution of the laser scars helps to confirm this.

(d)

Fluorescence: The ability of fluorescein to emit light of a longer wavelength (530 nm) when stimulated by light of a shorter wavelength (490 nm). Filters in the camera ensure blue light reaches the eye, and green-yellow light is captured on the film.

Blood–retinal barrier: Leakage of fluorescein dye is limited by the inner blood–retinal barrier (maintained by tight junctions between retinal capillary endothelial cells) and the outer blood–retinal barrier (maintained by tight junctions between retinal pigment epithelium cells).

(1 mark for each principle with explanation)

Feedback
The fundus fluorescein angiogram (FFA) is possible due to fluorescence, managed by appropriate filters in the camera, and blood–retinal barriers which govern the behaviour of intravenous fluorescein in the retinal and choroidal circulations.

Intravenous fluorescein is approximately 80% protein-bound, with the remainder being free fluorescein.

The endothelium of the retinal capillaries (the inner blood–retinal barrier) allows no leakage of fluorescein under normal circumstances. However, the choroidal capillaries (choriocapillaris) have a fenestrated endothelium which allows the passage of free fluorescein. This accounts for the normal diffuse patchy filling of the choroid seen before the retinal circulation fills. The outer blood–retinal barrier is formed by the tight junctions of retinal pigment epithelial cells, which prevents this free fluorescein from passing across to the neurosensory retina.

(e) Anaphylaxis

Feedback
Anaphylaxis to fluorescein is fortunately rare but can be life-threatening: the incidence of severe anaphylaxis is 1:1,900, and of fatal anaphylaxis is 1:220,000.

The risk of seizures is reported as 1:14,000.

(f) Any two of:
- Nausea and vomiting/gastrointestinal upset
- Yellow discolouration of urine/skin
- Flushing
- Itch
- Urticarial rash
- Pain at injection site due to extravasation

   (1 mark for each correct answer)

Feedback
These are more common, and usually mild side effects of fluorescein.

10. Answer

(a) Ophthalmia neonatorum (neonatal conjunctivitis)

(*1 mark for either nomenclature*)

Feedback
Ophthalmia neonatorum, also called neonatal conjunctivitis, is conjunctivitis affecting babies up to 1 month of age.

(b) *Neisseria gonorrhoeae*

Feedback
The Gram stain is negative (pink/red), and the electron micrograph of the organism shows diplococci. *Neisseria gonorrhoeae* is a Gram negative diplococcus and one of the two most important causes of ophthalmia neonatorum, the other being *Chlamydia trachomatis* (a Gram negative intracellular pathogen which has a coccoid or rod shape).

(c) Chocolate agar or Thayer–Martin medium (either acceptable)

Feedback
Chocolate agar is a non-selective growth medium whereas Thayer–Martin medium is selective for *Neisseria*.

(d) This is a sexually-transmitted infection that the baby acquires during passage through the birth canal.

Feedback
As neonatal conjunctivitis is usually acquired during birth, the date of onset can sometimes give a clue as to the organism responsible. Gonococcal conjunctivitis tends to present within the first few days of life and is notable for its severity, although other organisms, including *Chlamydia*, can present early too.

(e)
- Corneal scarring
- Perforation
- Endophthalmitis

(*1 mark each up to 2 marks*)

Feedback
Gonococcal conjunctivitis carries a significant risk of sight-threatening corneal involvement. This typically starts as a peripheral ulcer which may become ring-shaped, and if left untreated can cause corneal perforation or endophthalmitis.

(f) Systemic therapy

Feedback
The mainstay of treatment in neonatal conjunctivitis is systemic antibiotics, although topical antimicrobial therapy is often used as an adjunct. Gonococcal conjunctivitis can be treated with intravenous or intramuscular cephalosporin. Regular irrigation of the conjunctival sac is vital, and the baby's mother and her partner should be treated and undergo contact tracing.

(g) *Chlamydia trachomatis*

Investigations – any two of:
- Immunofluorescent staining (monoclonal antibody fluorescence microscopy)
- Polymerase chain reaction (PCR) or other nucleic acid amplification tests (NAAT)
- Enzyme-linked immunosorbent assay (ELISA)
- Culture
- Giemsa stain

(1 mark for correct organism, 1 mark each for two correct tests)

Feedback
Chlamydia is the most common cause of neonatal conjunctivitis.

The first three investigations listed can be performed on a conjunctival swab, and culture and Giemsa staining are ideally performed with a conjunctival scraping (due to *C. trachomatis* being an obligate intracellular pathogen).

Chlamydial conjunctivitis is usually treated with a 2–3 week course of oral erythromycin. Although it does not carry the same level of risk of sight-threatening corneal complications, it may cause systemic disease such as pneumonitis.

Other bacteria, such as *Staphylococcus aureus*, can cause neonatal conjunctivitis, and herpes simplex virus is a rare but serious cause.

11. Answer

(a)

Ray diagram of compound microscope

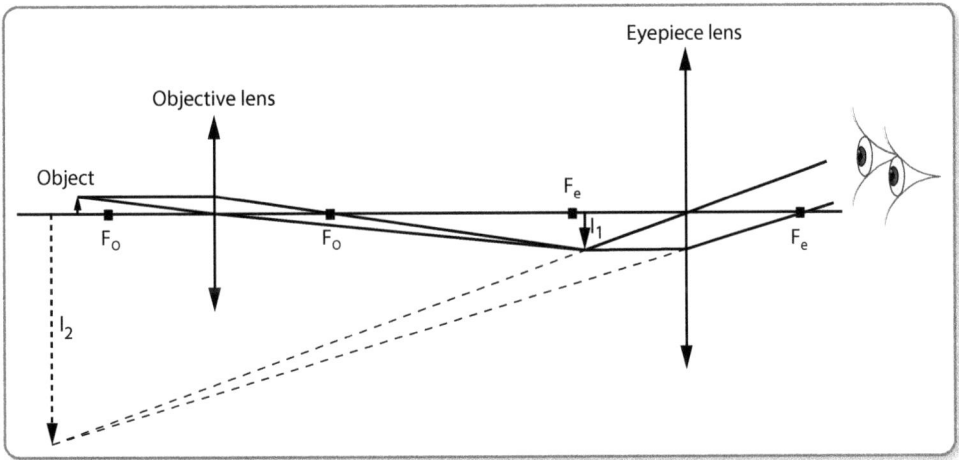

F_o = Principal focus of objective lens
F_e = Principal focus of eyepiece lens
I_1 = Image 1 (formed by objective lens), which acts as the object for the eyepiece lens. It is real, inverted and magnified
I_2 = Image 2 (formed by eyepiece lens), which is virtual, further magnified, 'erect' (i.e. remains inverted) and further from the lens than the object
(1 mark for each of the listed components, correctly drawn)

Feedback

The compound microscope consists of two lenses. The objective lens typically has the higher power of the two, and the object is placed very near it, just outside of its principal focus. The real, magnified, inverted image formed, image 1, then acts as the object for the eyepiece lens. However, this time the 'object' (image 1) falls within the principal focus and so the final image seen by the observer through the eyepiece lens is virtual, further magnified and remains inverted. Importantly, it is further from the eyepiece lens (and the observer) than image 1, which makes it easier to view.

(b)

Both the compound microscope and the astronomical telescope consist of two convex lenses and work on the same principles. The compound microscope uses a high-powered objective lens with the object near to its focal point to magnify very close objects. Conversely, the astronomical telescope uses a less powerful objective lens with a high-powered eyepiece lens, and magnifies very distant objects.

Also, in a compound microscope, the sum of the focal lengths is smaller than the distance between the lenses. In the astronomical telescope, the sum of the focal lengths is equal to the distance between the lenses.

(1 mark for similarities, 1 mark for differences)

Feedback

It is important not to confuse the astronomical (Keplerian) telescope with the Galilean telescope (which uses a high-powered concave eyepiece lens as opposed to the high-powered convex eyepiece lens of the astronomical telescope).

(c) Porro prism to invert the image, so that the final image is erect

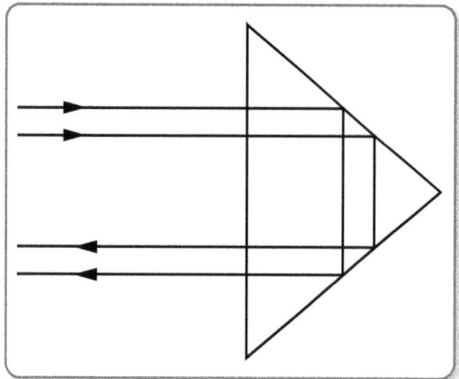

(1 mark for Porro prism, 2 marks for diagram)

(d) Two compound microscopes (one for each eye) are used, mounted at a 13–14° angle to each other.

Answers: CRQs

12. Answer

(a) A double-blind (double-masked) randomised controlled trial

[1 mark for double-blind (or double-masked), 1 mark for randomised controlled trial]

Feedback
In a randomised controlled trial, patients are randomly allocated to receive either the intervention or a placebo. The blinding refers to whether the patients or investigators are aware of which patients are receiving the intervention. Ideally both groups are 'blind' to which patients are receiving treatment, as this helps to avoid any bias. When this is the case the study is referred to as double-blind (double-masked is often the preferred term in ophthalmology trials).

You should be aware of a range of study designs, including meta-analyses, cohort studies, case-control studies, case series and case reports, and the hierarchy of evidence governing them.

(b)
The mean age is calculated as the sum of all the patients' ages in that arm divided by the number of patients. The median age is the age of the patient who is younger than half of the patients in that arm and older than the other half, i.e. the patient at the 50th percentile.

(1 mark for a reasonable definition of mean, 1 mark for a reasonable definition of median)

Feedback
You should be familiar with the calculation of mean, median and mode for a group. The mode of a group is the most frequently occurring value, so in this case would be the most frequently occurring age in the group.

(c) $33.\dot{3}\%$

Feedback
Relative risk reduction is the absolute risk reduction expressed as a percentage of the non-treatment risk. In this case the absolute risk reduction (the difference in the percentage risk between the two groups) is:

$$30\% - 20\% = 10\%$$

Therefore, the relative risk reduction is:

$$\frac{10}{30} \times 100 = 33.\dot{3}\%$$

(d) 10 patients

Feedback
The number needed to treat (NNT) is an expression of the number of patients that would need to be treated before one is likely to benefit from the treatment. It is calculated as the inverse of the absolute risk reduction (recall that the absolute

risk reduction is the difference in percentage risk between the two groups). In this case it would be:

$$\frac{1}{10\%} = \frac{1}{0.1} = 10$$

(e) That there is no difference in the recurrence rate of wet age-related macular degeneration (AMD) between the intervention group and the control group

or

That the recurrence rate of wet AMD is independent of whether a patient is receiving the new medication or a placebo.

Feedback
A null hypothesis proposes that there is no relationship between two measured variables. It is usually the objective of the study to attempt to disprove the null hypothesis. In this case the two measured variables that are key to the study are the recurrence rate of wet AMD and whether patients are receiving the treatment or a placebo, and therefore the null hypothesis is that there is no relationship between these two variables.

(f) A type I error is where the null hypothesis is rejected when it is true, i.e. a 'false positive'. In this study, a type I error would be concluding that the recurrence rate of wet AMD was dependent on whether or not a patient received the new treatment when in truth the new treatment did not affect the recurrence rate.

(1 mark for a general definition of a type I error, and 1 mark for describing a type I error in relation to this study)

Feedback
It is important to understand the definitions of type I and type II errors. A type I error is where the null hypothesis is rejected when it is true. A type II error is when a study fails to reject a null hypothesis when it is false (i.e. a 'false negative').

(g) The probability of the observed difference being due to chance is 4%.

Feedback
The P value is the probability of finding a difference at least as dramatic as that seen in the results as a chance occurrence. Recall that:

$$4\% = \frac{4}{100} = 0.04$$

It is usual practice for a study to set a significance level before undertaking statistical analysis (a P value below which it will be considered reasonable to reject the null hypothesis). This is usually 5% or 1% (i.e. $P \leq 0.05$ or $P \leq 0.01$).

EU GSPR Authorised Reprsentative
Logos Europe, 9 rue Nicolas Poussin
1700, La Rochelle, France
Phone: +33 (0) 6 67 93 73 78
E-mail: contact@logoseurope.eu

www.ingramcontent.com/pod-product-compliance
Ingram Content Group UK Ltd.
Pitfield, Milton Keynes, MK11 3LW, UK
UKHW050454150426
5217IPUK00025B/1684